SUCCESS IN ARTIFICIAL INSEMINATION - QUALITY OF SEMEN AND DIAGNOSTICS EMPLOYED

Edited by **Alemayehu Lemma**

Success in Artificial Insemination - Quality of Semen and Diagnostics Employed
http://dx.doi.org/10.5772/45731
Edited by Alemayehu Lemma

Contributors

Zahid Paksoy, Hüseyin Daş, Rita Payan Carreira, Paulo Borges, Fernando Mir, Alain Fontbonne, Alemayehu Lemma, Monteiro, Gustavo Guerino Macedo, Pietro Sampaio Baruselli, Joan E. Rodríguez-Gil, Daniel Tainturier, Mongkol Techakumphu, Nutthee Am-In, Wichai Tantasuparuk, Kakanang Buranaamnuay, Abelardo Silva Júnior, Carlos Eduardo Real Pereira, Eduardo Paulino da Costa, Emílio César Martins Pereira, Bakst, Jessica Dymond

Published by InTech

Janeza Trdine 9, 51000 Rijeka, Croatia

Publishing Process Manager Iva Simcic
Technical Editor InTech DTP team
Cover InTech Design team

Additional hard copies can be obtained from orders@intechopen.com

Success in Artificial Insemination - Quality of Semen and Diagnostics Employed , Edited by Alemayehu Lemma
p. cm.
ISBN 978-953-51-0920-4

For EU product safety concerns:
IN TECH d.o.o., Prolaz Marije Krucifikse Kozulić 3, 51000 Rijeka, Croatia,
info@intechopen.com or visit our website at intechopen.com.

Meet the editor

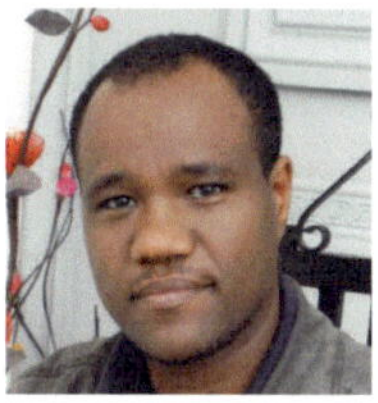

Alemayhu Lemma, DVM, PhD born in Ethiopia in January, 1967, graduated with DVM from Addis Ababa University (AAU) in 1990. He subsequently worked as a field veterinarian and later joined AAU in 1995. He completed his PhD studies in Animal Reproduction from Humboldt University of Berlin in 2004. Since then, he is working in the same university with continued researches in livestock reproduction mainly focusing on ovarian activities, AI, embryo transfer, and semen cryopreservation. He has authored/co-authored several scientific publications and contributed a chapter in a book on Artificial Insemination in farm Animals. He has over 20 years of expereince in veterinay science. He is currently head of the veterinary teaching hospital, and an associate professor in animal reproduction at AAU.

Contents

Preface

The extensive application of AI in domestic animals is demanding an efficient technique with high rate of success. Methods of improving the success of AI are subsequently emanating from continuous research in the areas of procuring the best quality semen that also require employing a rigours semen evaluation system. This book was prepared with an intention of creating a useful addition to an already available literature on different aspects of AI.

People involved in AI industry require up-to-date and relevant information in a more lucid and easily accessible way. Today, client education is increasingly becoming important and hence the mechanism to communicate pertinent research findings should only be through greater access to scholarly information. However, some of the most useful research findings published in scientific forums other than the common journals is still not accessible to all readers around the world. This is what makes InTech, as a pioneer open access publisher, an invaluable medium in meeting such needs.

Improvement in livestock resources can be achieved through the implementation of an efficient and reliable AI service, concomitantly with proper feeding, health care and management of livestock. Considering the economic investment in semen and other inputs, success must be judged on the basis of pregnancy rate to the first AI. Pregnancies resulting from AI largly originate from fertility level of the herd and semen quality. Collectively, errors in efficiency of AI result in high semen cost, poor conception rate, reduced cow production and net returns. An understanding of the impact of factors on the probability of success of AI is of primary importance to establish corrective measures. Despite the wide application and success of AI throughout the developed world, the success rate in many developing countries is still low.

The main objective of this book is to provide readers with scientific information on the role of high quality of semen in improving fertility and hence the success of AI. The book is divided in to ten chapters each addressing different aspects of AI in domestic animals. The first four chapters primarily focus on the importance of high semen quality in the success of AI and methods employed to improve semen quality. Research findings regarding the use of feed supplements in breeding animals, use of sex-sorted semen and modification of semen extenders in an attempt to improve semen quality have been dealt in detail. Chapters five and six address the female aspects including facts about the use anti-inflammatory drugs in the females, and the role of early pregnancy diagnosis in advancing the success rate of AI. Chapters seven through nine deals with aspects of advanced semen evaluation. Additional topic on AI in poultry has also been included. Totally over twenty-five authors and co-authors from different parts of the world have contributed to this work. Professional expertise from different continents, level of practices and interests have come together to produce a practicable compiled knowledge. This makes the book a valuable scholarly material for veterinarians working in AI industry, veterinary students, researchers and livestock practitioners.

Dr. Alemayehu Lemma
Department of Clinical Studies
Faculty of Veterinary Medicine
Addis Ababa University
Ethiopia

Chapter 1

The Importance of Semen Quality in AI Programs and Advances in Laboratory Analyses for Semen Characteristics Assessment

Leticia Zoccolaro Oliveira, Fabio Morato Monteiro,
Rubens Paes de Arruda and
Eneiva Carla Carvalho Celeghini

Additional information is available at the end of the chapter

http://dx.doi.org/10.5772/52022

1. Introduction

In the last decades, livestock sector has undergone a process of biotechnology incorporation with the main goal of enhancing productivity and improving the genetic makeup. In this sense, artificial insemination (AI) is considered as the most important biotechnology incorporated into livestock production systems because it implies the use and/or globalization of proven bulls, which represent a key tool in obtaining animals with higher genetic merit [1].

The wide use of bovine AI was mainly attributed to the development of methods that ensured cell viability after storage for long periods by reducing sperm metabolism, due to important progresses in studies involving cryoprotectants [2].

Nowadays, AI is considered as the most worldwide used reproductive biotechnology [3] with an extremely interesting benefit-cost relationship. Despite the unquestionable role of this biotechnology in improving productivity, many causes have accounted for the range in results and/or some unsatisfactory indices of bovine AI programs, highlighting several factors inherent to female physiology and/or farm management [4-9]. Nevertheless, another factor positively correlated with the AI outcomes that require appropriate attention, correspond to quality of semen samples used in the programs [10]. Therefore, the aim of this chapter is to review the importance of the quality of semen used in reproductive programs as well as the use of laboratory tests for predicting bull fertility.

2. The importance of semen quality for AI programs

Regarding the quality of semen used in AI programs, it has been reported that differences in fertility level could be attributed to variations in sperm qualitative characteristics [11].The success of bovine AI programs largely depends on the use of good quality semen. When only high fertility bulls are used, better conception rates are achieved, which reduces costs of reproductive programs [12].

Individual bulls may differ in their ability to fertilize oocytes and/or to develop to blastocyst stages after *in vitro* fertilization (IVF) procedures [12-18]. In addition, different sires and/or batches may differ in the individual response to induction of *in vitro* sperm capacitation methods, [14] and in the response to acrosomal mantainence after *in vitro* incubation [19].

Moreover, the bull influence is an important factor affecting *in vivo* reproductive outcomes [8,11, 20,21]. Ward et al. [20] demonstrated that kinetics of embryo development post insemination may vary between bulls. Andersson et al. [21] observed a high variability in fertility among bulls using different sperm concentrations per dose at AI. Sá Filho et al. [8] reported a high variation in conception rates depending on the bull utilized in a Timed-AI program. Moreover, Oliveira et al. [10] observed that the sire with numerically lower field fertility also presented inferior semen quality based on the several *in vitro* sperm characteristics assessed.

Furthermore, semen handling (and/or semen thawing protocol) might also be an important factor influencing in semen quality and, therefore, in AI results. Hence, it is deemed necessary to alert to the practice of simultaneous thawing of multiple semen straws at the moment of AI.

For instance, the Brazilian Association of Artificial Insemination recommends, for bovine AI, the thawing procedure of a single frozen semen straw (0.5 mL) in water bath unit at a temperature of 35 to 37°C for 30 seconds [22]. However, the large size of breeding herds using Timed-AI protocols in Brazil have resulted in the routine practice of thawing multiple straws simultaneously in the same water-bath unit to increase the convenience of semen handling and the number of inseminations in a short period.

Because the size of breeding herds continues to increase and the use of estrus synchronization (as well as the fixed-time artificial insemination protocols) becomes more frequent worldwide, there are increasing probabilities that several cows will be inseminated on the same day. Hence, several inseminators have used the practice of thawing, simultaneously, more than one straw of semen in the same thawing-bath unit to increase the convenience of semen handling. However, under these conditions, some straws remain in the thawing bath while insemination occurs. Consequently, the thermal environment of the water bath could have some influence in sperm viability and fertility.

With this concern Brown et al. [19] demonstrated, in a laboratory study, that semen straws must be agitated immediately after plunging to prevent direct contact among semen doses and refreezing during the thaw process. In this case, the simultaneous thawing of multiple straws had no effect on percentage of motile spermatozoa and acrosomal integrity when up to ten 0.5-mL semen straws were simultaneously thawed in a thermostatically controlled thawing bath of 36°C [19]. Later, several other studies were performed regarding this thawing practice, in order to evaluate the effect of simultaneous thawing of semen straws on *in vivo* fertility following AI [23-28].

Goodell [24], in a study with only 180 reproductive outcomes, reported a decrease in conception rates of the third and fourth insemination in the sequence, when more than two straws were thawed at once. However, Kaproth et al. [26] and Dalton et al. [27] demonstrated that experienced AI technicians can simultaneously thaw multiple semen straws and inseminate up to four cows within a 20 min interval, without adverse effects on field fertility. Sprenger et al. [25] observed that an interaction of herd by sequential insemination tended to influence field fertility outcomes. In one herd, conception rates of straws number 6 and ≥ 7 were lower than conception rates of straws 1 to 5. However, in the further eleven herds evaluated, sequential insemination had no effect on conception rate. The authors concluded that, given that recommended semen handling procedures are followed, more than two straws can be thawed at once without compromising semen fertility.

DeJarnette et al. [29,30] reviewed several studies regarding the effects of sequence of insemination after simultaneous thawing on conception rates with data collected from about 19,000 inseminations. The combined data from several studies suggested that several straws can be thawed at once with no significant fertility concern, provided that inseminators strictly adhere to recommended semen handling procedures. The authors recommended thawing (at 35°C for a minimum of 45 seconds) only the number of straws that can be deposited within 10 to 15 minutes in the female reproductive tract (always maintaining the thermal homeostasis during this interval) to avoid semen fertility impairment. In addition, it was stated that the more important issues regarding semen handling is time, temperature, hygiene and inseminator proficiency. Technicians that fail to abide by the standard recommendations will likely realize less than optimal conception rates irrespective of the number of straws thawed [29].

Hence, in general, the standard recommendations for cryopreserved bovine semen are (unless otherwise specified by the manufacturer): 1) to thaw no more straws than can be deposited in the female within 15 minutes between thawing and insemination, in a water-bath at 35°C for a minimum of 45 seconds, always maintaining thermal homeostasis during this interval; 2) Prevent direct straw to straw contact during the thaw process; 3) Implement appropriate thermal and hygienic protection procedures to maintain thermal homeostasis and cleanliness during gun assembly and transport to the cow [29].

Still, in a recent study, Oliveira et al. [28] observed that pregnancy rate was affected by sequence of insemination, depending on which bull was utilized in a timed AI program. In this experiment, groups of ten semen straws (0.5 mL) were simultaneously thawed at 36°C. After 30 seconds, semen straws were removed (one straw at a time) from water-bath and subsequently deposited in the cows for AI. One semen straw was used for each cow, in the same sequence that they were removed from water-bath. All animals utilized in the study were Nelore cows (n = 944). The inseminations were performed with semen from three Angus bulls, during Brazilian summer season (breeding season for beef cattle). Timed AI procedures were performed in a covered and protected area. The results demonstrated that one of the three sires had reduced fertility for inseminations performed with the group of straws associated with the longest interval from thawing to AI. However, semen from the other two bulls was not significantly different with respect to field fertility for any straw group (Straw Group 1: inseminations with 1st, 2nd and 3rd straws of the sequence; Straw Group 2: inseminations with 4th, 5th and 6th straws of the sequence; Straw Group 3: inseminations with 7th, 8th, 9th and 10th straws of the sequence). The mean time (±SD) of straws remaining in the thawing bath were 01:30 ± 00:51 for Straw Group 1, 03:36 ± 01:10 for Straw Group 2 and 06:13 ± 01:44 min for Straw Group 3. There was an interaction between sire and Straw Group (Conception rate of Sire 1: Straw Group 1 = 58.1%, Straw Group 2 = 60.2% and Straw Group 3 = 35.3%, $P < 0.05$; Conception rate of Sire 2: Straw Group 1 = 40.2%, Straw Group 2 = 50.5% and Straw Group 3 = 51.7%, $P > 0.05$; Conception rate of Sire 3: Straw Group 1 = 59.8%, Straw Group 2 = 51.0% and Straw Group 3 = 48.6%, $P > 0.05$). Overall conception rate of cows inseminated with first straw in the sequence (Straw 1) was 58% and of cows inseminated with tenth straw in the sequence (Straw 10) was 44% ($P > 0.05$). According to the results, semen fertility of some sires appeared to be more negatively affected by sequence of insemination than others. However, because the high environmental temperature during the field experiment may have potentiated the effects of incubation time on semen quality, the possibility that the thermal environment of thawing bath could have interfered on sperm fertility (mainly of bull that presented reduced conception rate associated to sequence of insemination), was considered. In summary, it was stated that the number of straws that can be simultaneously thawed without compromising semen fertility seems to vary for each bull. Unfortunately, the laboratory analyses did not clarified the effect of interaction between sire and straw group observed in field experiment of this respective study [28]. Thus, the reason why semen from some bulls seems to be more susceptible to specific thawing environments and/or procedures remained to be elucidated. The authors concluded that sequence of insemination after simultaneous thawing of multiple semen straws might affect fertility outcomes, depending on the sire utilized in the reproductive program. Hence, under similar environmental conditions, 10 semen straws should not be simultaneously thawed, because it could affect conception rates, according to the semen that is being used. Therefore, in similar routine procedures of timed AI programs consisting of large herds, it seems more cautious to not exceed the number of six semen straws for simultaneous thawing [28].

Similarly, Lee et al. [23] had previously reported that sequence of insemination may influence conception rates when up to four straws were thawed at once. Although all inseminations (n = 89) occurred within recommended time constraints (i.e., within the limit of 15 minutes between thawing to AI), the loaded AI guns were exposed to direct solar radiation (in a tropical environment; Hawaii) during transport from thawing-bath to cow. The data suggested that the thermal insult might had reflected in a linear reduction in conception rates from the first (48%) through the forth (25%) gun used in sequence [23].

Thus, an important consideration to be made is the possibility of a significant interaction between ambient temperature and interval to semen deposition. According to Shepard (unpublished; cited by [29]), an interaction of ambient temperature and interval to semen deposition might occur due to extended thaw duration (>10 min) when ambient temperatures are above 17°C, suggesting that higher environmental temperatures may be problematic to post-thaw fertility maintenance. In view of the fact that the studies of Lee et al. [23] and Oliveira et al. [28] were performed during warm seasons of tropical (or subtropical) environments, it can be suggested that greater sequences of insemination might compromise conception rates when associated with the effects of higher ambient temperatures and/or solar exposure.

Given the above observations, even though that many factors related to semen quality might influence AI outcomes, it is noteworthy that the use of high fertility bulls reduces the chances of field fertility impairment. Hence, an adequate evaluation of semen quality may reduce the effect of sire on reproductive outcomes, which is commonly observed in field trials. Thus, since a proper prediction of bull fertility is increasingly required, we consider appropriate to review the correlations between field fertility and *in vitro* sperm characteristics assessed by classical and modern semen analyses.

3. Correlation between *in vitro* sperm characteristics and *in vivo* bull fertility

Nowadays, many classical and modern methods have been used for laboratory assessment of *in vitro* semen characteristics following cryopreservation with the main purpose of predicting the fertility potential of a semen sample [11, 31-39].

Among the several sperm characteristics evaluated by laboratory techniques, sperm motility [33,40,41], morphology [42,43] and plasma membrane integrity [11,35,36,38] are the most used laboratory tests for assessing *in vitro* semen quality. However, the results of such assays do not always correlate with the real fertility of a semen sample [12,44].

In this sense, the relationship of *in vitro* semen characteristics and *in vivo* sire fertility has been the subject of much study [12,41,44,45-47]. Nevertheless, substantial variations are commonly observed in different experiments and low correlations are usually detected when single *in vitro* sperm characteristics are isolated compared to the field fertility [12,44]. Until now, the most efficient and accurate method to estimate the fertility of a particular bull is to accomplish the field fertility tests [44], which is very laborious, expensive and time consuming [46].

Alternatively, embryo culture techniques allow exploring *in vitro* bull fertility. The employment of such techniques has provided interesting but contradictory results regarding correlations between embryo *in vitro* embryo production (IVP) and *in vivo* bull fertility. Although positive correlations between IVP results and field fertility has been reported for some authors [12,14,16, 17, 20,46,48], other studies did not confirm the positive high correlations between *in vitro* fertilization (IVF) outcomes and *in vivo* fertility of evaluated sires [49,50,51]. However, Sudano et al. [12] recently demonstrated that it is possible to estimate bull fertility based on IVF outcomes, using a Bayesian statistical inference model.

Although interesting, it is still precipitated to ensure that the individual ability of fertilizing oocytes *in vitro* is a useful parameter for predicting *in vivo* bull fertility following AI. Hence, according to Ward et al. [20], a range of protocol variations among different IVP laboratories, the low repeatability in the results, as well as the various factors that may affect IVP outcomes, adds even more uncertainty if the *in vitro* ability for oocytes fertilization of a semen sample is sufficient accurate for predicting the sire field fertility. Additionally, it is noteworthy that more practical and/or simple laboratory techniques for assessing semen quality would be more advantageous for AI industry than the employment of IVP procedures.

Correa et al.[11] observed that the total number of motile spermatozoa tended to be higher in high fertility bulls. Farrell et al. [41] demonstrated that multiple combinations of motility sperm variables obtained by Computer Assisted Semen Analysis (CASA) had higher correlations with bull field fertility than single parameters evaluated separately. The authors observed that the combination of Progressive Motility, ALH (amplitude of lateral sperm head displacement), BCF (sperm beat cross frequency), and VAP (Average Path Velocity) presented high correlation value ($r^2 = 0.87$) and that the combination of ALH, BCF, linearity, VAP and VSL (Straight-Line Velocity) presented even higher correlation value ($r^2 = 0.98$). Hence, it has been demonstrated that sperm motility evaluations are important for the assessment of semen quality, mainly when CASA is used for assessing semen motility patterns. This non-subjective sperm analysis provides an opportunity to assess multiple characteristics on a large sample of spermatozoa, which allows assessing several sperm motility parameters with high repeatability [33,41].

Even though that computer-based analysis provides high accuracy of *in vitro* motility evaluation [33,41], the assessment of different aspects related to sperm physiology may guarantee better investigation of semen quality [38,52]. Changes in membrane architecture and sperm compartment functionality may interfere with cellular competence and with the process of fertilization. These changes can be monitored using fluorescent probes that are able to bind and stain specific structures of the cell permitting a direct diagnosis [38]. Celeghini et al. [38,53] reported an efficient and high-repeatability technique for simultaneous evaluation of the integrity of plasma and acrosomal membranes, as well as mitochondrial function, using a combination of the following probes: propidium iodide (PI), fluorescein isothiocyanate–Pisum sativum agglutinin (FITC-PSA) and tetrachloro-tetraethylbenzimidazolcarbocyanine iodide (JC-1) respectively.

Januskauskas et al. [35] found significant correlations between field fertility and plasma membrane integrity assessed by PI. Conversely, Brito et al. [54] reported no significant correlation between bovine *in vitro* fertilization (IVF) and plasma membrane integrity, measured by Eosin/Negrosin staining, CFDA/PI, SYBR-14/PI and HOST (hypo-osmotic swelling test). Nevertheless, Tartaglione and Ritta [36] demonstrated that the combination of plasma membrane integrity and functional laboratory tests presented high correlation coefficient with *in vitro* bull fertility. The authors demonstrated that combination of Eosin/Negrosin staining test with HOST presented high correlation coefficient with *in vitro* fertility outcomes. When sperm plasma and acrosomal membrane integrity results (assessed by Trypam/Blue Giemsa staining) were included in the regression model, a higher correlation coefficient was obtained. The authors emphasized that higher is the capacity for predicting semen fertility when higher number of sperm evaluations is performed [36].

Another concern of semen fertility studies is the occurrence of sperm oxidative stress. Spermatozoa are susceptible to oxidation of their plasma membranes due to the presence of polyunsaturated fatty acids [37]. Reactive oxygen species (ROS) may become cytotoxic through damage to proteins, nucleic acids and membrane lipids, if ROS concentrations overcome the natural defense mechanisms of the cell and extending medium [55]. Hence, since the high production of ROS might cause damages to plasma membrane structure, it can impair sperm function and motility [34,37]. A high degree of membrane lipid destabilization may lead to functional capacitation, reducing the sperm lifespan and fertilizing capacity [56]. In this sense, Hallap et al. [57] demonstrated that the amount of uncapacitated spermatozoa may provide valuable information about frozen–thawed semen quality.

Although the molecular basis involving the whole process of sperm capacitation has not yet been fully elucidated, it is recognized that sperm capacitation is a sequential event of biochemical alterations that involve numerous physiological changes. Some events related to the beginning of capacitation process include the removal of peripheral membrane factors, changes in membrane fluidity and in lipid composition [58,59]. Thus, the mammalian sperm capacitation is associated with reorganization of plasma membrane due to phospholipids redistribution of cholesterol removal [57]. Hence, the lipophilic probe Merocianina 540 may be used to monitor the level of phospholipid bilayer disorder of plasma membrane. Using this probe, the fluorescence intensity is increased with increasing membrane bilayer disorder, which can be an indicative of initial sperm capacitation process. In laboratory studies, this probe is commonly associated with the use of the probe Yo-Pro-1, which allows the simultaneous analysis of plasma membrane integrity. This is due to the fact that Yo-Pro-1 is a specific DNA probe with excitation and emission of fluorescence similar to the Merocianina 540 (around 540 nm) [57,58].

As stated above, oxidative stress is a recognized contributor to defective sperm function [34,37,39,60]. Spermatozoa is very susceptible to peroxidative damage because of their high cellular content of polyunsaturated fatty acids that are particularly vulnerable to this form of stress [37]. Recently, a fluorescence assay using the fluorophore 4,4-difluoro-5-(4-phenyl-1,3-butadienyl)-4-bora-3a,4a-diaza-s-indacene-3-undecanoic acid (C11-BODIPY$^{581/591}$) has been successfully applied for detecting lipid peroxide formation in living bovine sperm cells [34]. This assay relies on the sensitivity of C11-BODIPY$^{581/591}$, a fluorescent fatty acid conjugate, which readily incorporates into biological membranes [60]. Upon exposure to ROS, the C11-BODIPY$^{581/591}$ responds to free radical attack with an irreversible shift in spectral emission from red to green that can be quantified by flow cytometry [37,60]. Still, it is noteworthy that the negative effect of some ROS-generating systems does not require lipid peroxidation to induce cytotoxic changes in spermatozoa. In this sense, Guthrie and Welch [61] observed that Menadione and H_2O_2 decreased the percentage of motile sperm but had no effect on BODIPY oxidation.

In an interesting study, Kasimanickam et al. [39] reported that bull fertility was positively correlated to plasma membrane integrity and progressive motility. According to the authors, plasma membrane integrity significantly influenced the fertilizing capacity of a sire. Moreover, the authors demonstrated that plasma membrane integrity and progressive motility were negatively correlated to sperm lipid peroxidation and that lipid peroxidation and bull fertility was also high negatively correlated. Bulls with higher sperm lipid peroxidation were more likely to have a high DNA fragmentation and low plasma membrane integrity. Also, these bulls presented lower chances of siring calves [39]. These results are in accordance with Zabludovsky et al. [62] which also had demonstrated negative correlations between lipid peroxidation and IVF fertilization outcomes in humans.

It has frequently been reported that low-fertility bulls generally had high seminal content of morphologically abnormal cells [63]. Sperm with classically misshapen heads did not access the egg following AI since they do not traverse the female reproductive tract and/or participate in fertilization [43]. Some geometrical alterations of head morphology can cause differences in sperm hydrodynamics. According to [63], abnormal-shaped heads should be of primary concern regarding male fertility. The recognition of uncompensable cells in the ejaculate is currently best based on abnormal levels of sperm with misshapen heads [63].

Ostermeier et al. [32,64] also observed that some sperm morphometric variables were able to detect small differences in sperm nuclear shape which seems to be related to sire fertility. According to Beletti et al. [65], the application of computational image analysis for morphological characterization allows the identification of minor morphometric alterations of sperm head. However, little is known about the influence of such abnormalities on bull fertility. Because mammalian sperm heads consist almost entirely of chromatin, even minor changes in chromatin organization might affect sperm head shape. Nonetheless, morphological alterations in sperm head are not always caused by alterations in chromatin condensation. In the same way, chromatin abnormalities are not always followed by evident morphological irregularities [32,65,66].

A number of methods are available for identifying alterations in the stability of sperm chromatin. Sperm chromatin structure analysis (SCSA), currently the most used of these methods, is based on a flow cytometric evaluation of the fluorescence of spermatozoa stained with acridine orange [32,67]. Another method for chromatin evaluation uses a cationic dye, toluidine blue (at pH 4.0) that exhibits metachromasy. This dye binds to ionized phosphates in the DNA. In normal sperm chromatin, few dye molecules bind to DNA; this result in staining that varies from green to light blue. Spermatozoa with less compacted chromatin have more binding sites for the dye molecules, resulting in staining that varies from dark blue to magenta [65].

Whereas human-based methods for assessing sperm parameters involve a high degree of subjectivity in the visual analysis, computer-based methods for image processing and analysis are currently available. It can provide a more objective evaluation of cell motility and sperm morphological abnormalities, in addition to greater sensitivity, accuracy, speed and reproducibility. Computational morphometric analysis of spermatozoa usually considers basic measurements like the area, perimeter, length and width, as well as features derived from the measurements, such as the width:length ratio, shape factor and others [68]. An interesting approach is to use image analysis to characterize the sperm chromatin in smears stained with toluidine blue which also allows a morphometric analysis to be done concomitantly with the investigation of chromatin [65,69].

An interesting study of [32] demonstrated that the average of sperm head shape identified to be from high fertility bulls was more tapered and elongated (more elliptical) than the average shape of sperm identified to be from low fertility bulls. In addition, the authors observed that quantifying changes in sperm shape can be detected by Fourier parameters, which characterize the curvilinear perimeter of sperm head using harmonic amplitudes to describe the sperm nuclear shape. The relationship between sire fertility and Fourier parameters of sperm morphometric analysis was investigated. It was observed that Fourier descriptors were able to detect small differences in sperm nuclear shape from bulls with different fertility [32;64]. According to [63], the most promising method of quantifying changes in sperm head shape is utilizing the Fourier harmonic amplitude analysis.

Acevedo et al. [70] reported that spermatogenic disturbance resulted in production of abnormal sperm and that sperm DNA vulnerability to acid denaturation was positively associated with sperm having misshapen heads. This provided more support for the assertion that occurrence of sperm with misshapen heads can signal chromatin abnormalities and potential incompetence for fertilization of a semen sample [63]. Kasimanickam et al. [39] reported that some deleterious effects of sperm lipid peroxidation are also related to impairment in sperm DNA, which may also reduce bull fertilizing potential. The sires with high sperm DNA fragmentation index presented lower sperm fertilization potential; whereas sires with lower DNA fragmentation index presented higher chance of siring calves [39].

Besides the intense efforts from worldwide researchers, until now, no single laboratory test has accurately predicted the real fertilizing capacity of a semen sample [52, 71]. Hence, in spite of some interesting results of *in vitro* sperm characteristics, a notable consideration is the importance of field trials when definitive conclusions are taken regarding semen fertility.

4. Conclusions and implications

Individual bulls may differ in their ability to fertilize oocytes and/or to develop to blastocyst stages after *in vitro* and *in vivo* fertilization procedures. Hence, the success of bovine reproductive programs largely depends on the use of good quality semen. When only high fertility bulls are used, better fertilization rates and reproductives outcomes are achieved, increasing the reproductive efficiency and thus, reducing the costs of the programs.

The sequence of insemination after simultaneous thawing of multiple semen straws may present different effect and/or relevance on fertility outcomes, depending on the sire that is being used in the reproductive program. However, the reason why semen from some bulls seems to be more susceptible and/or differently affected to specific procedures, semen handling protocols, and/or environments remains to be further investigated. It is noteworthy, though, that the use of different sires, semen extenders, thawing bath volumes, semen straw volumes, AI technicians, semen handling procedures, number of AI guns utilized, ambient conditions, farm management and cow categories, as well as the use of different laboratory analyses, might generally influence the results obtained.

Worth mentioning though, that when the correct semen handling recommendation is provided, as well as the adequate cautious and/or proficiency of AI technician is assured, the sequence of insemination is not likely to severely impact semen quality and reproductive performance in AI programs. Thus, it is deemed reasonable to attempt to the fact that the care and concern with semen storage and handling is essential to obtain satisfactory reproductive outcomes after AI. In addition, greater attention should be directed to the simultaneous thawing of multiple semen straws, especially when the thawing procedures do not include a thermostatically controlled water-bath unit.

Even though that an *in vitro* semen assay for determining bull fertility would be of great benefit to AI programs, it is unlikely that the evaluation of a single sperm characteristic may reflect the real sperm fertilization capacity of a semen sample, considering the complexity of the reproductive process.

In spite of the promising results reported above, until now, no single laboratory test was able to accurately predict, with the required repeatability, the real fertilizing capacity of a sire. Hence, potential bull fertility can be estimated from laboratory semen assessment with higher accuracy when a combination of several *in vitro* sperm analysis is performed.

Still, further studies contributing to the understanding of seminal differences among bulls that might be related to differences in fertility rates commonly observed in AI programs must be encouraged.

Author details

Leticia Zoccolaro Oliveira[1], Fabio Morato Monteiro[2], Rubens Paes de Arruda[3] and Eneiva Carla Carvalho Celeghini[4]

1 Department of Animal Reproduction, FCAV, Univ Estadual Paulista, UNESP Jaboticabal, Jaboticabal, SP, Brazil

2 Animal Science Institute, IZ-APTA, Sertãozinho, SP, Brazil

3 Laboratory of Semen Biotechnology and Andrology, Department of Animal Reproduction, University of São Paulo, USP, Pirassununga, SP, Brazil

4 Department of Animal Reproduction, University of São Paulo, USP, São Paulo, SP, Brazil

References

[1] Sugulle AH, Bhuiyan MMU, Shamsuddin M. Breeding soundness of bulls and the quality of their frozen sêmen used in cattle artificial insemination in Bangladesh. Livestock Research for Rural Development 2006; 18 (4)1-10.

[2] Gao D, Mazur P, Crister J. Fundamental cryobiology of mammalian spermatozoa. In: Karow, A.M.; Critser, J.K. (eds.). Reproductive Tissue Banking. London: Academic Press, pp.263-328, 1997.

[3] Parkinson TJ. Evaluation of fertility and infertility in natural service bulls. The Veterinary Journal 2004; 168(1) 215–229.

[4] Bó GA, Baruselli PS, Martinez MF. Pattern and manipulation of follicular development in Bos indicus cattle. Animal Reproduction Science 2003; 78 (1) 307–326.

[5] Bó GA, Cutaia L, Peres LC, Pincinato D, Marana D, Baruselli PS. Technologies for fixedtime artificial insemination and their influence on reproductive performance of Bos indicus cattle. Society for Reproduction and Fertility 2007; .64(1) 223–236.

[6] Baruselli PS, Reis EL, Marques MO, Nasser LF, Bó GA. The use of hormonal treatments to improve reproductive performance of anestrous beef cattle in tropical climates. Animal Reproduction Science 2004; 82–83:.479–486.

[7] Perry GA, Smith MF, Roberts AJ, MacNeil MD, Geary TW. Relationship between size of ovulatory follicle and pregnancy success in beef heifers. Journal of Animal Science 2007; 85: 684-689.

[8] Sá Filho OJ, Meneghetti M, Peres R, Lamb G, Vasconcelos JLM. Fixedtime artificial insemination with estradiol and progesterone for Bos indicus cows. II. Strategies and factors affecting fertility. Theriogenology 2009; 72: 210–218.

[9] Bisinotto RS, Chebel RC, Santos JEP. Follicular wave of the ovulatory follicle and not cyclic status influences fertility of dairy cows. Journal of Dairy Science 2012; 93:.3578–3587.

[10] Oliveira LZ, Arruda RP, de Andrade AFC, Celeghini ECC, Santos RM, Beletti ME, Peres RFG, Oliveira CS, Hossepian de Lima VFM. Assessment of field fertility and several in vitro sperm characteristics following the use of different Angus sires in a timed-AI program with suckled Nelore cows. Livestock Science 2012; 146: 38–46.

[11] Correa JR, Pace MM, Zavos PM. Relationships among frozen thawed sperm characteristics assessed via the routine sêmen analysis, sperm functional tests and the fertility of bulls in an artificial insemination program. Theriogenology 1997; 48: 721-731.

[12] Sudano MJ, Crespilho AM, Fernandes CB, Martins Junior A, Papa FO, Rodrigues J, Machado R, Landim-Alvarenga F.C. Use of bayesian inference to correlate in vitro embryo production and in vivo fertility in Zebu bulls. Veterinary Medicine International 2011; ArticleID: 436381: 1-6.

[13] Hillery FL, Parrish JJ, First NL. Bull specific effect on fertilization and embryo development in vitro. Theriogenology 1990; 33, p.249.

[14] Marquant-Le Guienne B, Humblot P, Thibier M, Thibault C. Evaluation of bull sêmen fertility by homologous in vitro fertilization tests. Reproduction Nutrition Development 1990; 30: 259-266.

[15] Shi DS, Lu KH, Gordon I. Effects of bulls on fertilization of bovine oocytes and their subsequent development in vitro. Theriogenology 1990; 41: 1033–1043.

[16] Shamsuddin M, Larsson B. In vitro development of bovine embryos after fertilization using sêmen from different donors. Reproduction Domestic Animals 1993; 28: 77–84.

[17] Zhang BR, Larsson B, Lundeheim N, Rodriguez-Martinez H. Relationship between embryo development in vitro and 56-day nonreturn rates of cows inseminated with frozen-thawed sêmen from dairy bulls. Theriogenology 1997; 48: 221-231.

[18] Wei H, Fukui Y. Effects of bull, sperm type and sperm pretreatment on male pronuclear formation after intracytoplasmic sperm injection in cattle. Reproduction Fertility and Development 1999; 11: 59-65.

[19] Brown Jr DW, Senger PL, Becker WC. Effect of group thawing on post-thaw viability of bovine spermatozoa packaged in .5-milliliter French straws. Journal of Animal Science 1991; 69:.2303-2309.

[20] Ward F, Rizos D, Corridan D, Quinn K, Boland M, Lonergan P. Paternal influence on the time of first embryonic cleavage post insemination and the implications for subsequent bovine embryo development in vitro and fertility in vivo. Molecular Reproduction and Development 2001; .60: 47-55.

[21] Andersson M, Taponena J, Koskinena E, Dahlbomb M. Effect of insemination with doses of 2 or 15 million frozen-thawed spermatozoa and sêmen deposition site on pregnancy rate in dairy cows. Theriogenology 2004; 61: 1583-1588.

[22] CBRA - Colégio Brasileiro de Reprodução Animal. Manual para exame andrológico e avaliação de sêmen animal. 2. ed. Belo Horizonte, 1998.

[23] Lee CN, Huang TZ, Sagayaga AB. Conception rates in dairy cattle are affected by the number of sêmen straws thawed for breeding. Journal of Dairy Science 1997; 80 (Suppll), p.151.

[24] Goodell G. Comparison of AI pregnancy rates in dairy cattle by order of preparation of insemination straws. Journal of. Animal Science 2000; 78 (Suppl 1), p.229.

[25] Sprenger MJ, DeJarnette JM, Marshall CE. Conception rates of sequential inseminations after batch-thawing multiple straws of sêmen: A professional technician case study. Journal of Animal Science 2001;.79 (Suppl 1): p.253.

[26] Kaproth MT, Parks JE, Grambo GC, Rycroft HE, Hertl JA, Gröhn YT. Effect of preparing and loading multiple insemination guns on conception rate in two large commercial dairy herds. Theriogenology 2002; 57: 909-921.

[27] Dalton JC, Ahmadzadeh A, Shafii B, Price WJ, DeJarnette JM. Effect of simultaneous thawing of multiple 0.5-mL straws of sêmen and sequence of insemination on conception rate in dairy cattle. Journal of Dairy Science 2004; 87: 972-75.

[28] Oliveira LZ, Arruda RP, de Andrade AFC, Santos RM, Beletti ME, Peres RFG, Martins JPN, Hossepian de Lima VFM. Effect of sequence of insemination after simultaneous

thawing of multiple semen straws on pregnancy rate to timed AI in suckled multiparous Nelore cows. Theriogenology 2012; 78 (8): 1800-1813.

[29] DeJarnette JM, Shepard RW, Kaproth MT, Michael NA, Dalton JC, Goodell GM, Lee CN. Effects of sequential insemination number after batch-thawing on conception rates of cryopreserved bovine semen: a review. In: Proceeding of the 19th Technical Conference on Artificial Insemination and Reproduction. Columbia, MO, USA. p.102-108, 2002.

[30] DeJarnette JM, Marshall CE, Lenz RW, Monke DR. Sustaining the Fertility of Artificially Inseminated Dairy Cattle: The Role of the Artificial Insemination Industry. Journal of. Dairy Science 2004; 87: E93–E104.

[31] Revell SG, Mrode RA. An osmotic resistance test for bovine sêmen. Animal Reproduction Science 1994; 36: 77-86.

[32] Ostermeier GC, Sargeant GA, Yandel BS, Evenson DP, Parrish JJ. Relationship of bull fertility to sperm nuclear shape. Journal of Andrology 2001; 22: 595–603.

[33] Verstegen J, Iguer-Ouada M, Oclin K. Computer assisted sêmen analyzers in andrology research and veterinary pratice. Theriogenology 2002; 57: 149-179.

[34] Brouwers JF, Gadella BM. In situ detection and localization of lipid peroxidation in individual bovine sperm cells. Free Radical Biology and Medicine 2003; 35: 1382–1391.

[35] Januskauskas A, Johannisson A, Rodriguez-Martinez H. Subtle membrane changes in cryopreserved bull sêmen in relation with sperm viability, chromatin structure and field fertility. Theriogenology 2003; 60: 743-758.

[36] Tartaglione CM, Ritta MN. Prognostic value of spermatological parameters as predictors of in vitro fertility of frozen-thawed bull sêmen. Theriogenology 2004; 62 (7): 1245–1252.

[37] Aitken R, Wingate J, De Iullis G, Mclaughlin E. Analysis of lipid peroxidation in human spermatozoa using BODIPY C11. Molecular Human Reproduction 2007; 13: 203-211.

[38] Celeghini ECC, Arruda RP, De Andrade AFC, Nascimento J, Raphael CF. Practical techniques for bovine sperm simultaneous fluorimetric assessment of plasma, acrosomal and mitochondrial membranes. Reproduction Domestic Animals 2007; 42:.479–488.

[39] Kasimanickam R, Kasimanickam V, Thatcher CD, Nebel RL, Cassell BG. Relationships among lipid peroxidation, glutathione peroxidase, superoxide dismutase, sperm parameters, and competitive index in dairy bulls. Theriogenology 2007; 67: 1004–1012.

[40] Kjaestad H, Ropstad E, Berg KA. Evaluation of spermatological parameters used to predict the fertility of frozen bull sêmen. Acta Veterinaria Scandinavica 1993; 34 (3): 299–303.

[41] Farrell PB, Presicce GA, Brockett CC, Foote RH. Quantification of bull sperm characteristics measured by computer-assisted sperm analysis (CASA) and the relationship to fertility. Theriogenology 1998; 49: 871-879.

[42] Barth AD. The relationship between sperm abnormalities and fertility. In: Proceedings of the 14th Technical Conference on Artificial Insemination and Reproduction, NAAB, Columbia, MO, pp.47–63, 1992.

[43] Saacke RG, DeJarnette JM, Bame JH, Karabinus DS, Whitman S. Can spermatozoa with abnormal heads gain access to the ovum in artificially inseminated super- and single-ovulating cattle? Theriogenology 1998; 51:117–128.

[44] Zhang BR, Larsson B, Lundeheim N, Haard MGH, Rodriguez-Martinez H. Prediction of bull fertility by combined in vitro assessments of frozen-thawed sêmen from young dairy bulls entering an Al-programme. International Journal of Andrology 1999; 22: 253–260.

[45] Amann RP. Can the fertility potential of a seminal sample be predicted accurately? Journal Andrology 1989; 10: 89-98.

[46] Larsson B, Rodrıguez-Martınez H. Can we use in vitro fertilization tests to predict sêmen fertility? Animal Reproduction Science 2000; 60-61: 327–336.

[47] Rodriguez-Martinez H. Laboratory sêmen assessment and prediction of fertility: still Utopia? Reproduction Domestic Animals 2003; 38: 312–318.

[48] Lonergan P. The application of in vitro fertilization techniques to the prediction of bull fertility. Reproduction Domestic Animals 1994; 29: 12-21.

[49] Schneider CS, Ellington JE, Wright RW. Relationship between bull field fertility and in vitro embryo production using sperm preparation methods with and without somatic cell co-culture. Theriogenology 1999; 51 (6): 1085–1098.

[50] Papadopoulos S, Hanrahan JP, Donovan A, Duffy P, Boland MP, Lonergan P. In vitro fertilization as a predictor of fertility from cervical insemination of sheep. Theriogenology 2005; 63 (1): 150–159.

[51] Vandaele L, Mateusen B, Maes D, de Kruif A, van Soom A. Is apoptosis in bovine in vitro produced embryos related to early developmental kinetics and in vivo bull fertility? Theriogenology 2006; 65 (9): 1691–1703.

[52] Arruda RP, Celeghini ECC, Alonso MA, Carvalho HF, Oliveira LZ, Nascimento J, Silva DF, Affonso FJ, Lemes KM, Jaimes J.D. Métodos de avaliação da morfologia e função espermática: momento atual e desafios futuros. Revista Brasileira Reprodução Animal 2011:35 (2); 145-151.

[53] Celeghini ECC, Arruda RP, De Andrade AFC, Nascimento J, Raphael CF, Rodrigues PHM. Effects that bovine sperm cryopreservation using two different extenders has on sperm membranes and chromatin. Animal Reproduction Science 2008; 104: 119–131.

[54] Brito LFC, Barth AD, Bilodeau-Goeseels S, Panich PL, Kastelic JP. Comparison of methods to evaluate the plasmalemma of bovine sperm and their relationship with in vitro fertilization rate. Theriogenology 2003; 60:.1539-1551.

[55] Storey, B.T.Biochemistry of the induction and prevention of lipoperoxidative damage in human spermatozoa. Molecular Human Reproduction., v.3, p.203–213, 1997.

[56] Mortimer SJ, Maxwell WMC. Effect of medium on the kinematics of frozen-thawed ram spermatozoa. Reproduction 2004; 127: 285-291.

[57] Hallap T, Nagy S, Jaakma U, Johannisson A, Rodriguez-Martinez H. Usefulness of a triple fluorochrome combination Merocyanine 540/Yo-Pro 1/Hoechst 33342 in assessing membrane stability of viable frozen-thawed spermatozoa from Estonian Holstein AI bulls. Theriogenology 2006; 65: 1122–1136.

[58] Saravia F, Hernández M, Wallgren M, Johannisson A, Rodríguez-Martínez H. Controlled cooling during sêmen cryopreservation does not induce capacitation of spermatozoa from two portions of the boar ejaculate. International Journal of Andrology 2007; 30,(6): 485-499.

[59] Gadella BM. Sperm membrane physiology and relevance for fertilization. Animal Reproduction Science 2008; 107: 229-236.

[60] Neild DM, Brouwers JF, Colenbrander B, Aguero A, Gadella BM. Lipid peroxide formation in relation to membrane stability of fresh and frozen thawed stallion spermatozoa. Molecular Reproduction and Development 2005; 72: 230–238.

[61] Guthrie HD, Welch GR. Use of fluorescence-activated flow cytometry to determine membrane lipid peroxidation during hypothermic liquid storage and freeze-thawing of viable boar sperm loaded with 4, 4-difluoro-5-(4-phenyl-1,3-butadienyl)-4-bora-3a, 4a-diaza-s-indacene-3-undecanoic acid. Journal of Animal Science 2007;85:1402-11.

[62] Zabludovsky N, Eltes F, Geva E, Berkovitz E, Amit A, Barak Y, Har-Even D, Bartoov B. Relationship between human sperm lipid peroxidation, comprehensive quality parameters and IVF outcome. Andrologia 1999; 31: 91–98.

[63] Saacke RG. Sperm morphology: Its relevance to compensable and uncompensable traits in sêmen. Theriogenology 2008; 70: 473–478.

[64] Ostermeier GC, Sargeant GA, Yandel BS, Parrish JJ. Measurement of bovine sperm nuclear shape using the Fourier harmonic amplitudes. Journal of Andrology 2001; 22: 584–594.

[65] Beletti ME, Costa LF, Guardieiro MM. Morphometric features and chromatin condensation abnormalities evaluated by toluidine blue staining in bull spermatozoa. Brazilian Journal of Morphological Sciences 2005; 22: 85–90.

[66] Beletti ME, Costa LF, Viana MP. A comparison of morphometric characteristics of sperm from fertile Bos taurus and Bos indicus bulls in Brazil. Animal Reproduction Science 2005; 85:.105–116.

[67] Evenson DP, Larson KL, Jost LK. The sperm chromatin structure assay (SCSA): clinical use for detecting sperm DNA fragmentation related to male infertility and comparisons with other techniques. Journal of. Andrology 2002; 23: 25-43.

[68] Garrett C, Baker HW. A new fully automated system for the morphometric analysis of human sperm heads. Fertility and Sterility 1995; 63: 1306-1317.

[69] Beletti ME, Costa LF. A systematic approach to multi-species sperm morphometrical characterization. Analytical and Quantitative Cytology and Histology 2003; 25: 97–107.

[70] Acevedo NJ, Bame H, Kuehn LA, Hohenboken WD, Evenson DP, Saacke RG. Sperm chromatin structure assay (SCSA) and sperm morphology. In: Proceedings of the 19th Technical Conference on Artificial Insemination and Reproduction, National Association of Animal Breeders, Columbia, MO, p. 84–90, 2002.

[71] Arruda RP, de Andrade AFC, Peres KR, Raphael CF, Nascimento J, Celeghini ECC. Biotécnicas aplicadas à avaliação do potencial de fertilidade do sêmen equino. Revista Brasileira Reprodução Animal 2007, 31 (1) 8-16.

Chapter 2

Improvement of Semen Quality by Feed Supplement and Semen Cryopreservation in Swine

Mongkol Techakumphu, Kakanang Buranaamnuay,
Wichai Tantasuparuk and Nutthee Am-In

Additional information is available at the end of the chapter

http://dx.doi.org/10.5772/51737

1. Introduction

Artificial insemination in pig offers many advantages in swine production in terms of a better disease control through semen quality control, a diverse male genetic distribution and an easiness of management. It is accepted that in developing countries, AI helps to improve the genetic profile. A number of sows can be inseminated using the same ejaculate instead of only one from natural mating. The number of pig farms using AI has increased because of the technical improvement of semen extenders and equipments, and the technique can be performed on farm. In Thailand, AI in commercial pig farms is routinely used as a standard protocol in pig production. The results obtained by AI are quite similar or higher than that from natural. Because of the quality of insemination can be guaranteed by semen testing and evaluation before insemination. The improvement of semen quality can be acquired by feed supplement and semen freezing in boar can be used to genetic conservation. The feed supplement improving the semen quality have been imperatively used in the boars which have low libido and low semen quality, because these boars have been imported and are of superior genetic merit and so are perceived to have great value to their owners who, therefore, are very reluctant to cull them. Moreover, in tropical countries, cryopreservation of boar semen is nowadays performed in a limited scale and it has yet to be conducted in Thailand particularly for the commercial purpose. Concerning this point and obtained benefit in the future, the improvement of boar semen quality by feed supplement and boar semen cryopreservation are reviewed in this chapter.

2. Feed supplement to increase boar semen quality

The semen quality depends on individual, breed, season, confinement and boar health. It was found that the dietary supplements of antioxidants, vitamins and/or minerals can increase libido and semen characteristics in boars. Additions of antioxidants in seminal plasma or semen extender play an important role on boar semen storability. Semen with a normal motility contains higher polyunsaturated fatty acids (PUFAs) in cell membrane has that that having a low motility [1]. Short life span spermatozoa usually presented in low antioxidant condition resulting from the high lipid peroxidation of sperm plasma membrane. Spermatozoa in low antioxidants of seminal plasma also show a lower sperm motility, viability and normal morphology than spermatozoa in normal seminal plasma (Table 1) [1,2]. The feed supplements were expected to improve the semen quality by increasing the number of sperm per ejaculation, motility, viability and antioxidant in cell and seminal plasma. However, it depends on the initial performance of the boar influencing on successfully improving semen quality. Therefore, the key roles of feed supplement containing the rich of PUFAs, vitamins and minerals to improve the semen quality are increasing the antioxidant to reduce the plasma membrane damages from ROS and increase the amount of PUFAs in sperm plasma membrane that may increase the percentage of sperm motility and vitality.

3. Effect of Reactive Oxygen Species (ROS)

Boar sperm are highly sensitive to peroxidative damage due to the high content of unsaturated fatty acids in the phospholipids of the sperm plasma membrane [3,4] and the correlation of low antioxidant capacity of boar seminal plasma and lipid-peroxidation [5]. It has been reported in sperm freezing of human [6], bull [7] and mouse [8] that is associated with ROS level and oxidative stress. Moreover, the process of freezing and thawing bovine spermatozoa can generate the ROS [9], DNA damage [10], cytoskeleton alterations [11], inhibition of the sperm–oocyte fusion [12] and can affect the sperm axoneme that is influenced on the sperm motility [13].

The lipid-peroxidation of membrane phospholipid bound docosahexaenoic acid (DHA) has been presented as one of the major factors that limit the sperm motility in vitro. Semen samples show high sperm variability in lifespan and, consequently, in susceptibility toward lipid peroxidation. Therefore, it is postulated that there is also cell-to-cell variability in DHA content in human spermatozoa and that the content of the main substrate of lipid peroxidation (DHA) is critical and highly regulated during the sperm maturation process. Several studies have been performed to analyze the fatty acid content of germ cells and sperm at different stages of maturation, including in vivo studies in animal models, and in vitro approaches in human spermatozoa. One of the consequences of defective sperm maturation in the seminiferous epithelium is the retention of residual cytoplasm. This residual cytoplasm, which is attached to the midpiece and retronuclear area of the sperm head, has been shown to produce high levels of reactive oxygen species (ROS) [14-16]. In addition, the membranes enclosing the residual cytoplasm are enriched in polyunsaturated fatty acids such as DHA [17,18]. The combination of high polyunsaturated fatty acid content and high ROS production in these immature sperm has been shown to lead to increased lipid peroxidation and subsequent loss of sperm function [14,15]. ROS-mediated damage to human spermatozoa was characterized in the early 1980s [19-24] and has been shown by many authors to be an important factor in the pathogenesis of male infertility [14,25-27].

To a first approximation, the process of lipid peroxidation involves the initial abstraction of a hydrogen atom from the bis-allylic methylene groups of polyunsaturated fatty acids, mainly DHA, by molecular oxygen. This leads to molecular rearrangement to a conjugated diene and addition of oxygen, resulting in the production of lipid peroxide radical. This peroxyradical can now abstract a new hydrogen atom from an adjacent DHA molecule leading to a chain reaction that ultimately results in lipid fragmentation and the production of malonaldehyde and toxic shortchain alkanes (e.g., propane). These propagation reactions are mediated by oxygen radicals. DHA is the major polyunsaturated fatty acid in sperm from a number of mammalian species, including the human, accounting in this species for up to 30% of phospholipid-bound fatty acid and up to 73% of polyunsaturated fatty acids. At the same time, DHA is the main substrate of lipid peroxidation, accounting for 90% of the overall rate of lipid peroxidation in human spermatozoa [23,28].

Characteristics	Normal motility	Low motility
Sperm per ejaculate ($\times 10^{9}$)	88.6 ± 41.7^{a}	76.9 ± 36.2^{a}
Sperm motility, %	82.6 ± 5.2^{a}	30.6 ± 12.8^{b}
Sperm viability, %	86.7 ± 5.8^{a}	31.5 ± 14.9^{b}
Normal morphology, %	96.2 ± 1.9^{a}	85.1 ± 4.9^{b}
Normal plasma membrane, %	83.3 ± 7.4^{a}	15.7 ± 7.5^{b}
Total antioxidant status in seminal plasma (ng/ml)	1.54 ± 0.35^{a}	0.80 ± 0.56^{b}

Rows with different superscripts (a,b) differ P≤0.05 [1-2]

Table 1. Semen characteristics and antioxidant capacity in seminal plasma of boars having normal and low sperm motility (means ± SD)

Lipid peroxidation has profound consequences in biological membranes. The generation of the polar lipid peroxides ultimately results in the disruption of the membrane hydrophobic packing, inactivation of glycolytic enzymes, damage of axonemal proteins (loss of motility), acrosomal membrane damage, and DNA alterations [29,30]. Oxidation of phospholipid-bound DHA has been shown to be the major factor that determines the motile lifespan of sperm in vitro [6,31,32]. Three basic factors determine the overall rate of lipid peroxidation of sperm in vitro: oxygen concentration and temperature in the medium (OXIDANT), the presence of antioxidant defenses (ANTIOXIDANT), and the content of membrane-bound DHA (SUBSTRATE). Thus, the higher the temperature and the concentration of oxygen in solution, the higher the rate of lipid peroxidation as measured by malonaldehyde production [24]. In boar, total antioxidant in seminal plasma relates to percentage of normal sperm morphology and plasma membrane. The low storability semen has presented the high plasma membrane damage from ROS, which was resulted from low amount of antioxidant in seminal plasma [2]. Moreover, the semen which having poor normal sperm morphology has shown the low level of antioxidant in seminal plasma (Table 1) [1].

The balance between these key factors determines the overall rate of peroxidation in vitro. In this system, the substrate seems to play a key role. The main substrates for lipid peroxidation are polyunsaturated fatty acids, especially docosahexaenoic acid.

4. Effect of vitamins and minerals

The glutathione peroxidase is main intracellular antioxidant enzyme that catalyses to reduce the hydrogen peroxide and organic hydroperoxides to nontoxic metabolized compounds. The essential component of this enzyme is selenium. Vitamin E or alpha-tocopherol is the dominant antioxidant in cell plasma membranes. Many researches have shown a synergism of antioxidant activity between selenium in glutathione peroxidase and vitamin E. The effects of selenium supplementation on semen quality were more reported than the effects of vitamin E supplementation, and selenium supplementation improved in higher conception rates when gilts were serviced with extended semen from the boars [33]. However, feed additive on boar diet with high levels of vitamin C had no effects on semen quality or libido characteristics in healthy boars. U.S. Food and Drug Administration (FDA) regulations allow up to 136 g of selenium add on/pound of feed for pigs.

Vitamin C or ascorbic acids are a dominant water-soluble antioxidant. Their action is scavenger to disable the function of any type ROS. Vitamin C is a powerful source of electron donor which reacts with hydroxyl radicals, peroxide and superoxide to form de-hydroxyl ascorbic acid. The level of ascorbic acid in seminal plasma is approximately 10-fold higher concentration comparing with blood plasma in human [30,34]. The level of ascorbic acid in seminal plasma has a positively correlation with the percentage of normal [35].

5. Effect of Polyunsaturated Fatty Acids (PUFAs)

Linoleic acid or omega-6 fatty acid is the only FA for which NRC has established requirements at least 0.1% of diet for sexually active boars. However, the effect of various fatty acids (FAs) top on diet, particularly the omega-3 fatty acids, on semen quality and libido characteristics in boars are more interesting. Nowadays, there are 3 types of omega-3 fatty acids that are linolenic, eicosapentaenoic (EPA) and docosahexaenoic (DHA). The boar feed commonly consist of the large amounts of crops, with source of protein added in the form of soya-bean, fish powder, bone powder, etc. Thus, dietary fatty acids have a (n-6):(n-3) normal ratio of greater than 6:1 and do not contain long chain n-3 PUFAs. If 22:6(n-3) is essential for optimal fertility in pig spermatozoa, as being in human sperm [28,36,37], then it is possible that supplement 22:6(n-3) PUFAs on boar diets to improve the spermatogenesis. This supplementation may increase from either a deficit of (n-3) fatty acids or an increasing synthesis of 22:6(n-3) from 18:3(n-3) to competition between (n-6) and (n-3) fatty acids [38]. The tuna oil supplementing on the boar diet can increase the percentages of sperm cells with progressive motility, the proportion of live sperm, normal acrosome head, and normal morphology [39]. It was found that boars fed withcommercially available product containing DHA, vitamin E and selenium (PROSPERM®, Minitube America, Inc., Minneapolis, MN) for 16 weeks had a higher sperm concentration, number of sperm/ejaculate, and sperm motility comparing with control group [40]. In many experiments, 8-week period was used as the control period because spermatogenesis in boars requires 34–39 d and epididymal transport involves another 9–12 d [41]. It is not surprising that a 7–8 week period may be necessary after dietary supplementation [40,42].

6. Boar semen cryopreservation

The research on semen cryopreservation in boar is limited even though the procedures have been studied during the past 60 years [43-47]. The advantages for development of frozen semen include the preservation of the good genetic resource, the distribution of superior genetic boars, and the improvement of the transportation of sperm across countries [48]. However, the utilization of frozen-thawed (FT) semen prepared for artificial insemination (AI) at present is estimated to be less than 1% of all insemination worldwide. The most important reasons are the poor sperm quality after cryopreservation and a lower fertilizing capacity of FT semen, when used for conventional AI compared to fresh semen. Poor sperm quality frequently found in FT boar semen is partly due to a high sensitivity of the boar sperm to rapid cooling to a few degrees above 0C, the so-called "cold shock", which the sperm have to traverse during cryopreservation process. This is evidenced by the loss of viable sperm and by more capacitation-like changes in the viable sperm [49]. These changes result in a shorter survival time of the FT sperm in the female genital tract in comparison to its fresh and liquid-preserved counterparts [50,51].

7. Factors affecting the success of boar semen cryopreservation

Boar semen differs in several respects from the semen of other domestic animals. It is produced in large volume (200 to 250 ml) and is extremely sensitive to cold shock. The success of freezing boar semen depends on both internal and external factors. Internal factors include the inherent characteristics of sperm and the existing differences among boars and ejaculates, while external factors are composed of the composition of the extenders, freezing packages, and the method of freezing and thawing of the semen, for example [48].

8. The semen donors

Variation between individuals in the extent to which their sperm are damaged by freeze-thawing has been reports in many species including pig [52-55]. For instance, some study assigned individual boars into good, average and poor freezability groups on the basis of their post-thaw sperm viability using a system of multivariate pattern analysis, and suggested that cryosurvival of the sperm was not necessarily related to the observed quality of the semen sample. In addition to inter-animal variation, intra-animal variation such as difference between ejaculate fractions has also been described as a source of difference in boar sperm freezability [56,57]. Some researcher found that sperm present in the first 10 ml of the sperm-rich fraction (portion I) better sustain cooling and freeze-thawing compared to those present in the rest of the ejaculate (portion II) [56]. These differences were manifested by motility patterns, the maintenance of membrane integrity and capacitation-like changes of sperm after thawing. However, variation between ejaculate fractions is dependent of individual boars, with some boars differing in the ability of the two ejaculate portions to sustain cryopreservation, while in other boars such differences were not detected [57]. The mechanisms underlying differences in cryosensitivity between different individuals and different ejaculate portions have yet to be elucidated, but there is some evidence for physiological differences between sperm from individual boars. Harrison and co-workers demonstrated that the stimulatory effects of bicarbonate on the process of capacitation differ among individual boars [58]. Also, the existence of differences in seminal plasma composition and sperm morphology has been hypothesized as a possible explanation for the distinct ability of different boars and different ejaculate portions to sustain cryopreservation [59,60]. In general, boar sperm heads present in portion I were significantly shorter and wider than those present in portion II, detected by using computer-assisted sperm head morphometry analysis (ASMA) [57]. It has been hypothesized that such differences could be genetic in origin. Thurston and co-workers using Amplified fragment length polymorphism (AFLP) technology to analyze genome of 22 Yorkshire (Y) boars indicated that 16 candidate genetic markers linked to genes controlling sperm freezability and these genomes varied among individual boars. Consequently, they may be useful for the prediction of both post-thaw semen quality and fertility of individual boars [55].

9. The composition of freezing extenders

A number of substances have been added to boar semen during cryopreservation in order to improve FT sperm quality. It has been investigated that egg yolk added to boar semen could protect sperm acrosomes during cold shock and hence reduce cryodamage of FT boar sperm [61]. Protection has been claimed to be due to both phospholipids and the low density lipoprotein fraction in egg yolk [62,63]. The mechanism of action is unclear but could be mediated by either a less intense cellular dehydration or by stabilization of the sperm plasma membrane [51].

Cryoprotective agents (CPAs) have been divided into those that penetrate the cell and those which remain extracellular. Glycerol considered as penetrating agents and other non-penetrating agents such as various sugars have been evaluated for cryoprotective effect in boar sperm [64,65]. Glycerol in low concentrations (3 to 4%) has been utilized in various techniques of sperm cryopreservation [47,66]. At these concentrations, glycerol gives maximum post-thaw viability and also in vitro fertilizing capacity of sperm [43]. Both post-thaw motility and acrosome integrity of boar sperm would be decreased when glycerol concentration reached 5%. Glycerol and other penetrating agents could improve FT sperm survival by penetrating sperm and reduce the shrinkage of the cells developed during cooling [8]. They could also lower the freezing point of extra-cellular fluid via action of non-penetrating CPAs [67]. Therefore, the damage of sperm from the formation of intracellular ice occurred during freezing is reduced.

The success of the boar sperm cryopreservation was dramatically increased when the detergent Sodium Dodecyl Sulphate (SDS; later known as Equex STM paste) was included in the cryopreservation protocol [68,69]. The addition of SDS to semen extenders decreases freeze-thaw damage to sperm in several species, including boar [70-72]. Pursel and co-workers stated that the use of 0.5% Orvus Es Paste, a commercial preparation of SDS, in the BF5 extender significantly enhanced the preservation of fertilizing capacity concomitant with an increase in post-thaw percentages of normal acrosome morphology and motility of boar sperm [69]. The beneficial effect of SDS on the sperm membrane is not fully understood, but it has been suggested that its protective effect is mediated through a change in the extending medium, by solubilization of the protective lipids in the egg yolk contained in the extenders. This effect enhanced the cold shock resistance of sperm [73,74]

10. Freezing packages

Boar sperm have been frozen in many forms of packages. Pellet, a form of freezing bull semen on dry ice, was adapted to freeze boar semen and first reported as in [47]. Boar sperm have also been frozen in 5-ml maxi-, 0.5-ml medium- and 0.25-ml mini-straws, as well as different types of 5-ml flat plastic bags [67,75]. All package forms have their own advantages and drawbacks. The 5-ml maxi-straw contains one insemination dose but has a relatively small surface-to-volume ratio, which constrains optimal freezing and thawing throughout the sample. The plastic bags allow even more homogeneous freezing and thawing and also contain a whole insemination dose, but they are not suited for storage in standard liquid nitrogen containers, and therefore are not in commercial use [71]. Pellets and the small straws (0.25- and 0.5-ml straws) have a cryobiologically suitable shape with a large surface-to-volume ratio; thus theoretically, FT sperm in pellets and small straws are less damaged than those in maxi-straws [76,77]. However, with pellets, there are difficulty in the identification of the doses and a risk of cross-contamination during storage, and the thawing procedure is rather complicated as well [71]. Also, the small packages could contain relatively few sperm such as 250 to 500 x10^6 sperm per straw, which are not enough for a single dose of conventional AI in pigs. Eriksson and Rodriguez- Martinez developed a new flat plastic container (the FlatPack®) for freezing boar semen. This package could contain a complete insemination dose, allows a quick and uniform freezing and thawing due to its large surface-to-volume ratio, and fits into any conventional liquid nitrogen container. Nonetheless, insemination with large numbers of sperm, such as 5 to $6x10^9$ sperm per dose, reduces the number of AI doses per ejaculate. Achieving successful AI with fewer sperm is more important if using boars of superior genetic merit [71].

Fertility after transcervial deep AI of FT boar semen.

11. Conventional AI in pigs

Three techniques of AI can be performed by conventional, intrauterine and deep intrauterine. The conventional AI is commen in fresh semen practice, while intrauterine with a reduce concentration of semen is increasing with a satisifying result. The deep intrauterine insemination is used for special kind of semen such as frozen semen or sexed semen with a reduce and semen can be deposited near the junction of uterine-oviductal junction.

Conventional AI in domestic pigs is practiced with doses of approximately $3x10^9$ sperm extended to a volume of 80 to 100 ml. Semen doses are stored at temperatures ranging 16 to 20°C, usually for up to 3 days in simple extenders, but longer when using other extenders [78,79]. The semen is deposited into the posterior region of the cervix by using a disposable, often an intra-cervical, catheter whose tip stimulates the corkscrew shape of the boar penis and engages with the posterior folds of the cervix as it occurs during natural mating. In general, the AI process starts 12 h after detection of standing estrus and it is repeated every 12 to 18 h until standing estrus is no longer shown. When proper detection of estrus is performed, the farrowing rate (FR) and litter size (LS) are comparable with those achieved by natural mating, reaching over 90% of FR and mean LS of 14 piglets [80].

12. Use of FT semen in porcine AI

Contrary to what occurs in cattle, where FT semen is routinely used for AI [81], cryopreserved boar semen is used in less than 1% of the AIs performed around the world. The reasons behind this restricted use of FT boar semen are the low survivability of sperm after the freeze-thawing process and the shorter lifespan of the surviving sperm. These result in lower FR and small LS compared with AI using semen preserved in liquid form [48]. Furthermore, owing to the restricted lifespan of the FT boar sperm, excessive sperm numbers are used often 5 to 6 $x10^9$ sperm per dose. Moreover, at least two AIs are usually performed per estrus in order to reach acceptable fertility rates in the field [82]. Altogether, few doses can be obtained from a single ejaculate and too many sperm are used to ensure fertilization. A decrease in the number of sperm per dose is therefore required to improve the use of ejaculates, so that the production will be cheaper and the use of genetically superior sires more effective.

13. Transcervical deep AI

Although few sperm are required for fertilization within the oviduct, this reduced number is the product of a sequential and very effective reduction along the process of sperm transport in the female reproductive tract (i.e., 25 to 40% of inseminated sperm are lost with the backflow and 50% of the rest of the sperm are ingested by leukocytes in the uterus; Matthijs et al., 2003). The problem to be overcome during AI is to get an adequate number of sperm to the uterotubal junction (UTJ) that could ensure the establishment of the functional sperm reservoir with enough viable, potentially-fertile sperm to ensure maximal fertilization. One strategy proposed to accomplish this is to decrease the number of sperm per AI-dose, by depositing the semen directly in the uterus, and get sufficient sperm into the UTJ. Such deep AI with reduced sperm numbers is a relatively new reproductive practice that has attracted the attention of the swine industry. Such a method could also be advantageous for the spreading of AI with FT semen.

There are basically two non-surgical procedures for depositing sperm into the pig uterus. These include semen deposition either in the uterine body [49,75,83] or into the uterine horn [84,85].

Intra-uterine insemination (IUI) (Figure 1a)

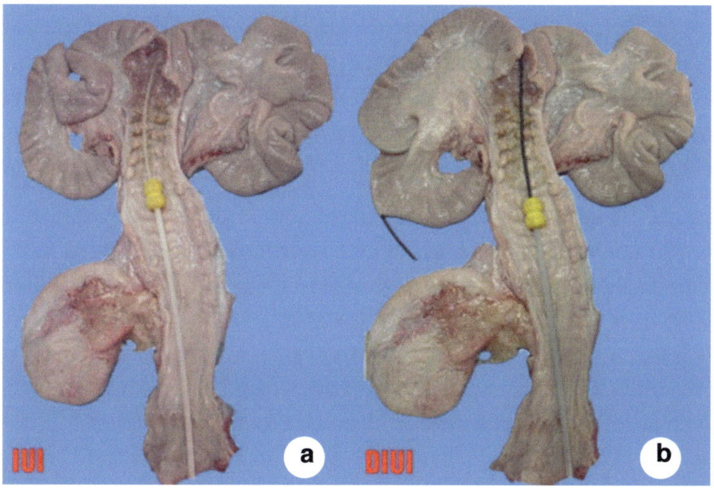

Figure 1. Sperm can be deposited in different procedures: (a) intra-uterine insemination (IUI) and (b) deep intra-uterine insemination (DIUI)

A non-traumatic transcervical catheter that allows an easy penetration of the cervix and deposition of semen in the uterine body of the sow has been designed. Briefly, a conventional catheter (outer catheter) is placed toward and locked into the cervix. An inner tube (around 4 mm outer diameter) is passed through the outer catheter, along the cervical lumen, to reach the uterine body or the posterior part of one of the uterine horns (about 200 mm beyond the tip of the outer catheter). The IUI catheter can be used with minimal training and it does not seriously delay the process of insemination, although it can only be safely used in sows [83]. Under commercial conditions, use of the IUI catheter with extended fresh semen can reduce sperm numbers to $1x10^9$ sperm per insemination dose and results in a comparable effect on both FR and LS (89% FR and 12 LS) compared with 91% FR and 12.5 LS after conventional AI with $3x10^9$ sperm. However, in the field trials carried out by references [86,87], FR were similar between IUI with $1x10^9$ sperm and conventional AI with $3x10^9$ sperm, but IUI sows had significantly less piglets born per litter (1.5 to 2 smaller LS). The reasons for the loss in LS have not been clarified. Rozeboom and co-workers suggested that several factors such as aged sperm, improper semen handling or insemination-ovulation interval can cause decreases in reproductive performances when low numbers of sperm are used, and in order to obtain consistently high fertility results, a slightly higher number of sperm should be considered.

14. Deep intra-uterine insemination (DIUI) (Figure 1b)

Non-surgical DIUI has been performed in non-sedated pigs using a flexible fiber optic endoscope (1.35 m length, 3.3 mm outer diameter) inserted via the vagina and cervix to reach the upper segment of one uterine horn [84]. The procedure required 3 to 5 min in 90% of the females. After this DIUI, only 1% of the sows showed signs of uterine infection. However, the endoscope is a highly expensive instrument and unpractical for routine use. A flexible catheter was therefore developed on the basis of the propulsion force and flexibility of the fibro-endoscope [85]. The method allows deposition of low sperm doses of either fresh or FT sperm. Moreover, the technology can be successfully used to produce piglets with sex-sorted sperm [88], or for embryo transfer [89].

Using fresh semen, FR and LS were not statistically different between DIUI with $150x10^6$ sperm per dose and conventional AI with $3x10^9$ sperm, ranging from 83 to 87% FR and 9.2 to 10.4 LS [88]. Nonetheless, LS was always lowest in the DIUI sows. Similarly, although no differences in FR were found (83% and 90% for DIUI and conventional AI, respectively), DIUI sows had less LS (10.5 and 12.9, respectively). The low LS achieved in the DIUI sows inseminated with $150x10^6$ sperm probably resulted from the high incidence of unilateral or incomplete bilateral fertilization, and could be overcome by increasing the number of inseminated sperm to $600x10^6$ sperm per dose [90]. On the other hand, when a single DIUI with $150x10^6$ sperm was performed in hormonally induced ovulating sows, both FR and LS of DIUI sows (83% and 9.7) were not different from those of conventional AI sows (83% and 10) [85]. When FT semen ($1x10^9$ sperm per dose) was used for DIUI, promising results were obtained. With hormonally induced ovulation and a single DIUI, the FR was 77.5% and LS was 9.3, while with spontaneous ovulation and two DIUIs, the FR was 70% and LS was 9.3. The lower fertility obtained in the latter group resulted from the suboptimal insemination-ovulation period [91]. Bolarin and staff working with spontaneously ovulating sows (n=407) obtained FR of over 80% and about 10 piglets born per litter when two DIUIs, at 6 h interval, with only $1x10^9$ FT sperm per dose were conducted at the peri-ovulatory period [92]. It has been suggested that DIUI should be carried out ≤ 8 h before spontaneous ovulation when FT sperm are used [93].

15. Boar semen cryopreservation, experiences in Thailand

In tropical countries including Thailand, cryopreservation of boar semen is nowadays performed in a very limited scale and it has yet to be conducted for the commercial purpose. Our studies undertaken between 2004 and 2009 therefore aimed to develop boar semen cryopreservation in Thailand. Effects of straw volume, Equex STM paste added to a freezing extender and of the individual differences on boar sperm quality after cryopreservation were investigated. In addition, in vivo fertility results such as fertilization rate, FR and LS of FT boar semen after DIUI and IUI in multiparous sows were evaluated.

Using a lactose-egg yolk extender with 9% glycerol as a freezing extender of boar semen, it was demonstrated that after thawing the motility, viability and NAR of sperm evaluated with conventional methods were improved when 1.5% Equex STM paste was added into the freezing media [94]. This finding confirms beneficial effects of the detergent on preventing/diminishing cell damage during the freeze-thawing process [68,95]. Equex STM paste improves post-thaw survival of sperm by acting as a surfactant to stabilize cell membranes, particularly acrosomal membranes, and to protect sperm against the toxic effects of glycerol during cryopreservation [73]. However, since the positive effects of this substance are only observed in the present of egg yolk in the semen extender, it is suggested that Equex STM paste exerts its beneficial action through the alteration of low-density lipoproteins in egg yolk rather than directly affects sperm membranes [69].

In theory, post-thaw sperm loaded in 0.5-ml straws which have smaller surface-to-volume ratio should not have a better quality than those in 0.25-ml straws. Nevertheless, based on the results of 12 ejaculates from 4 boars evaluated in our study [94], the viability and normal morphology of FT sperm packaged in 0.5-ml straws were superior to those in 0.25-ml straws despite being frozen and thawed with their own optimal protocols. The reason behind this is unknown, but it is interesting that similar results have also been observed in dog semen [96]. Therefore, in order to find the reason and draw conclusions with boar sperm, more investigations in this aspect might have to be performed.

With regard to effect of individual variations on the FT sperm quality, 45 ejaculates of 15 boars from three breeds (Landrace (L), Y and Duroc (D); 5 boars each) were studied [97]. It was found that the breed of boar and the individual boars within the same breed significantly influenced most of the FT sperm parameters evaluated. For instance, the post-thaw sperm viability in D and L boars was significantly higher than Y boars. The motility and the normal morphology of FT sperm were lowest in Y boars. L boars seemed to have the most variations in many of the FT sperm parameters. The difference in sperm quality among individual boars that was found in our study was in agreement with previous findings [52,98], suggesting that such individual variation may be correlated with difference in physiological characteristic of the sperm plasma membrane among boars. Additionally, the genomic differences between individual boars may be responsible for freezability and post-thaw quality of their sperm [55].

Cervical AI with FT semen usually results in suboptimal fertility; thereby, deep AI using IUI and DIUI procedures was developed. We evaluated fertility (fertilization rate, FR and LS) of FT boar semen after IUI, with $2x10^9$ total sperm per dose, and DIUI, with $1x10^9$ per dose, in spontaneously ovulating weaned sows. The results revealed that at approximately 2 days following inseminations either with IUI or DIUI, embryo(s) could be recovered from both sides of the oviducts. This observation, the first report in FT semen [99], was consistent with previous studies where the extended fresh semen was used [85,100,101]. It was demonstrated that both transuterine and transperitoneal migrations were involved in transport of sperm inseminated using DIUI to reach the other side of the oviduct [85]. Nonetheless, comparing between techniques, fertilization rate in the IUI group was significantly higher than the DIUI group. The reason for this finding might not associate with the insemination techniques, but rather it was a result of insemination time relative to the moment of ovulation which was not appropriate in the DIUI group (≥ 8 h before ovulation).

After AI using the same procedures (IUI and DIUI) and same numbers of FT sperm (1 to 2 $x10^9$ per dose), acceptable fertility (67% FR and 7.7 to 10.5 LS) were obtained in both groups ($P>0.05$); however, TB in the DIUI group was about 3 piglets fewer than the IUI group. This was probably the consequence of inadequate numbers of functional sperm used for DIUI ($400x10^6$ motile sperm) which leaded to the unilateral and/or incomplete bilateral fertilization and resulted in the low LS [102] (Table 2)

	Insemination procedure	
	IUI	**DIUI**
No. of sows	9	9
Parity number (mean±SD)	5.0±1.9	4.8±1.9
Weaning to estrus interval (days) (mean±SD)	4.9±0.9	5.1±1.5
Sows inseminated within 6 h before/after ovulation (%)	8/9 (89)	9/9 (100)
Non-return rate at 24 days (%)	8/9 (89)	6/9 (67)
Sows return-to-estrus after 24 days (%)	2/8 (25)	0 (0)
Farrowing rate (%)	6/9 (67)	6/9 (67)
Number of total piglets born per litter (mean±SD)	10.5±2.9	7.7±3.0
Number of piglets born alive per litter (mean±SD)	9.5±3.0	7.5±3.0

Table 2. Non-return rate, farrowing rate, number of total piglets born per litter and number of piglets born alive per litter after intra-uterine insemination (IUI) and deep intra-uterine insemination (DIUI) with frozen-thawed boar semen [102]

According to the results of our studies, it could be indicated that timing of insemination in relation to ovulation and sperm numbers per insemination dose are important factors for successful insemination regardless of insemination procedures and types of semen used. The time of insemination factor becomes more essential when using FT semen because the life span of FT sperm in the female reproductive tract is relatively short compared with the fresh cells, i.e. 4 to 8 h vs about 24 h after insemination, respectively [103,104]. It has been demonstrated that the number of sperm per insemination dose is related to both the number of functional sperm colonized in the oviductal sperm reservoir and fertilization rate [49,101]. Insufficient sperm numbers in the DIUI group might account for the lower fertilization rate [99] and thus smaller LS [102].

16. Conclusion

The feed supplement containing the rich of PUFAs, vitamins and minerals can improve the sperm motility, vitality and number of sperm per ejaculation in boar. The success of feed supplement depends on the initial performance of the boar. They may not improve the semen quality if the boars are the good performance of semen producers. Moreover, taking all of our researches, we can conclude that the production of cryopreserved boar semen and AI with FT boar semen could be successfully performed in Thailand and its application in commercial farm is undergoing. An IUI procedure was considered to be suitable for FT boar semen to produce acceptable fertility rates. This is very useful for the conservation and/or production of animal with high genetic merits.

Author details

Mongkol Techakumphu[1*], Kakanang Buranaamnuay[2], Wichai Tantasuparuk[1] and Nutthee Am-In[1]

1 Department of Obstetrics Gynaecology and Reproduction, Faculty of Veterinary Science, Chulalongkorn University, Thailand

2 Institute of Molecular Biosciences (MB), Mahidol University, Thailand

References

[1] Am-in N, Kirkwood RN, Techakumphu M, Tantasuparuk W. Lipid profiles of sperm and seminal plasma from boars having normal or low sperm motility. Theriogenology 2011;75: 897-903.

[2] Am-in N, Kirkwood RN, Techakumphu M, Tantasuparuk W. Effect of storage for 24 h at 18C on sperm quality and a comparison of two assays for sperm membrane lipid peroxidation. Can J Anim Sci 2010;90: 389-392.

[3] Cerolini S, Maldjian A, Surai P, Noble R. Viability, susceptibility to peroxidation and fatty acid composition of boar semen during liquid storage. Anim Reprod Sci 2000;58: 99-111.

[4] Parks JE, Graham JK. Effects of cryopreservation procedures on sperm membranes. Theriogenology 1992;38: 209-222.

[5] Brezezinska-Slebodzinska E, Slebodzinski AB, Pietras B, Wieczorek G. Antioxidant effect of vitamin E and glutathione on lipid peroxidation in boar semen plasma. Biol Trace Elem Res 1995;47: 69-74.

[6] Alvarez JG, Storey BT. Evidence for increased lipid peroxidative damage and loss of superoxide dismutase activity as a mode of sublethal cryodamage to human sperm during cryopreservation. J Androl 1992;13: 232-241.

[7] O'Flaherty C, Beconi M, Beorlegui N. Effect of natural antioxidants, superoxide dismutase and hydrogen peroxide on capacitation of frozen-thawed bull spermatozoa. Andrologia 1997;29: 269-275.

[8] Mazur P, Katkov, II, Katkova N, Critser JK. The enhancement of the ability of mouse sperm to survive freezing and thawing by the use of high concentrations of glycerol and the presence of an Escherichia coli membrane preparation (Oxyrase) to lower the oxygen concentration. Cryobiology 2000;40: 187-209.

[9] Chatterjee S, Gagnon C. Production of reactive oxygen species by spermatozoa undergoing cooling, freezing, and thawing. Mol Reprod Dev 2001;59: 451-458.

[10] Lopes S, Jurisicova A, Sun JG, Casper RF. Reactive oxygen species: potential cause for DNA fragmentation in human spermatozoa. Hum Reprod 1998;13: 896-900.

[11] Hinshaw DB, Sklar LA, Bohl B, Schraufstatter IU, Hyslop PA, Rossi MW, Spragg RG, Cochrane CG. Cytoskeletal and morphologic impact of cellular oxidant injury. Am J Pathol 1986;123: 454-464.

[12] Aitken RJ, Clarkson JS, Fishel S. Generation of reactive oxygen species, lipid peroxidation, and human sperm function. Biol Reprod 1989;41: 183-197.

[13] de Lamirande E, Gagnon C. Reactive oxygen species and human spermatozoa. I. Effects on the motility of intact spermatozoa and on sperm axonemes. J Androl 1992;13: 368-378.

[14] Aitken J, Krausz C, Buckingham D. Relationships between biochemical markers for residual sperm cytoplasm, reactive oxygen species generation, and the presence of leukocytes and precursor germ cells in human sperm suspensions. Mol Reprod Dev 1994;39: 268-279.

[15] Gil-Guzman E, Ollero M, Lopez MC, Sharma RK, Alvarez JG, Thomas AJ, Jr., Agarwal A. Differential production of reactive oxygen species by subsets of human spermatozoa at different stages of maturation. Hum Reprod 2001;16: 1922-1930.

[16] Gomez E, Buckingham DW, Brindle J, Lanzafame F, Irvine DS, Aitken RJ. Development of an image analysis system to monitor the retention of residual cytoplasm by human spermatozoa: correlation with biochemical markers of the cytoplasmic space, oxidative stress, and sperm function. J Androl 1996;17: 276-287.

[17] Huszar G, Vigue L. Incomplete development of human spermatozoa is associated with increased creatine phosphokinase concentration and abnormal head morphology. Mol Reprod Dev 1993;34: 292-298.

[18] Ollero M, Powers RD, Alvarez JG. Variation of docosahexaenoic acid content in subsets of human spermatozoa at different stages of maturation: implications for sperm lipoperoxidative damage. Mol Reprod Dev 2000;55: 326-334.

[19] Alvarez JG, Holland MK, Storey BT. Spontaneous lipid peroxidation in rabbit spermatozoa: a useful model for the reaction of O2 metabolites with single cells. Adv Exp Med Biol 1984;169: 433-443.

[20] Alvarez JG, Storey BT. Spontaneous lipid peroxidation in rabbit epididymal spermatozoa: its effect on sperm motility. Biol Reprod 1982;27: 1102-1108.

[21] Alvarez JG, Storey BT. Assessment of cell damage caused by spontaneous lipid peroxidation in rabbit spermatozoa. Biol Reprod 1984;30: 323-331.

[22] Alvarez JG, Storey BT. Lipid peroxidation and the reactions of superoxide and hydrogen peroxide in mouse spermatozoa. Biol Reprod 1984;30: 833-841.

[23] Alvarez JG, Storey BT. Differential incorporation of fatty acids into and peroxidative loss of fatty acids from phospholipids of human spermatozoa. Mol Reprod Dev 1995;42: 334-346.

[24] Alvarez JG, Touchstone JC, Blasco L, Storey BT. Spontaneous lipid peroxidation and production of hydrogen peroxide and superoxide in human spermatozoa. Superoxide dismutase as major enzyme protectant against oxygen toxicity. J Androl 1987;8: 338-348.

[25] Aitken J, Fisher H. Reactive oxygen species generation and human spermatozoa: the balance of benefit and risk. Bioessays 1994;16: 259-267.

[26] de Lamirande E, Gagnon C. Reactive oxygen species (ROS) and reproduction. Adv Exp Med Biol 1994;366: 185-197.

[27] Sharma RK, Agarwal A. Role of reactive oxygen species in male infertility. Urology 1996;48: 835-850.

[28] Zalata AA, Christophe AB, Depuydt CE, Schoonjans F, Comhaire FH. The fatty acid composition of phospholipids of spermatozoa from infertile patients. Mol Hum Reprod 1998;4: 111-118.

[29] Alvarez JG, Sharma RK, Ollero M, Saleh RA, Lopez MC, Thomas AJ, Jr., Evenson DP, Agarwal A. Increased DNA damage in sperm from leukocytospermic semen samples as determined by the sperm chromatin structure assay. Fertil Steril 2002;78: 319-329.

[30] Fraga CG, Motchnik PA, Shigenaga MK, Helbock HJ, Jacob RA, Ames BN. Ascorbic acid protects against endogenous oxidative DNA damage in human sperm. Proc Natl Acad Sci U S A 1991;88: 11003-11006.

[31] Aitken RJ, Harkiss D, Buckingham D. Relationship between iron-catalysed lipid peroxidation potential and human sperm function. J Reprod Fertil 1993;98: 257-265.

[32] Jones R, Mann T, Sherins R. Peroxidative breakdown of phospholipids in human spermatozoa, spermicidal properties of fatty acid peroxides, and protective action of seminal plasma. Fertil Steril 1979;31: 531-537.

[33] Marin-Guzman J, Mahan DC, Chung YK, Pate JL, Pope WF. Effects of dietary selenium and vitamin E on boar performance and tissue responses, semen quality, and subsequent fertilization rates in mature gilts. J Anim Sci 1997;75: 2994-3003.

[34] Lewis SE, Sterling ES, Young IS, Thompson W. Comparison of individual antioxidants of sperm and seminal plasma in fertile and infertile men. Fertil Steril 1997;67: 142-147.

[35] Thiele JJ, Friesleben HJ, Fuchs J, Ochsendorf FR. Ascorbic acid and urate in human seminal plasma: determination and interrelationships with chemiluminescence in washed semen. Hum Reprod 1995;10: 110-115.

[36] Conquer JA, Martin JB, Tummon I, Watson L, Tekpetey F. Fatty acid analysis of blood serum, seminal plasma, and spermatozoa of normozoospermic vs. asthenozoospermic males. Lipids 1999;34: 793-799.

[37] Nissen HP, Kreysel HW. Polyunsaturated fatty acids in relation to sperm motility. Andrologia 1983;15: 264-269.

[38] Sprecher H. Interactions between the metabolism of n-3 and n-6 fatty acids. J Intern Med Suppl 1989;731: 5-9.

[39] Rooke JA, Shao CC, Speake BK. Effects of feeding tuna oil on the lipid composition of pig spermatozoa and in vitro characteristics of semen. Reproduction 2001;121: 315-322.

[40] Strzezek J, Fraser L, Kuklinska M, Dziekonska A, Lecewicz M. Effects of dietary supplementation with polyunsaturated fatty acids and antioxidants on biochemical characteristics of boar semen. Reprod Biol 2004;4: 271-287.

[41] Swierstra EE. Cytology and duration of the cycle of the seminiferous epithelium of the boar; duration of spermatozoan transit through the epididymis. Anat Rec 1968;161: 171-185.

[42] Estienne MJ, Harper AF, Crawford RJ. Dietary supplementation with a source of omega-3 fatty acids increases sperm number and the duration of ejaculation in boars. Theriogenology 2008;70: 70-76.

[43] Almlid T, Johnson LA. Effects of glycerol concentration, equilibration time and temperature of glycerol addition on post-thaw viability of boar spermatozoa frozen in straws. J Anim Sci 1988;66: 2899-2905.

[44] Bamba K, Cran DG. Effect of rapid warming of boar semen on sperm morphology and physiology. J Reprod Fertil 1985;75: 133-138.

[45] Crabo B, Einarsson S. Fertility of deep frozen boar spermatozoa. Acta Vet Scand 1971;12: 125-127.

[46] Fiser PS, Fairfull RW. Combined effect of glycerol concentration and cooling velocity on motility and acrosomal integrity of boar spermatozoa frozen in 0.5 ml straws. Mol Reprod Dev 1990;25: 123-129.

[47] Pursel VG, Johnson LA. Freezing of boar spermatozoa: fertilizing capacity with concentrated semen and a new thawing procedure. J Anim Sci 1975;40: 99-102.

[48] Johnson LA, Weitze KF, Fiser P, Maxwell WM. Storage of boar semen. Anim Reprod Sci 2000;62: 143-172.

[49] Watson PF. The causes of reduced fertility with cryopreserved semen. Anim Reprod Sci 2000;60-61: 481-492.

[50] Pursel VG, Schulman LL, Johnson LA. Distribution and morphology of fresh and frozen-thawed sperm in the reproductive tract of gilts after artificial insemination. Biol Reprod 1978;19: 69-76.

[51] Watson PF. Recent developments and concepts in the cryopreservation of spermatozoa and the assessment of their post-thawing function. Reprod Fertil Dev 1995;7: 871-891.

[52] Holt WV, Medrano A, Thurston LM, Watson PF. The significance of cooling rates and animal variability for boar sperm cryopreservation: insights from the cryomicroscope. Theriogenology 2005;63: 370-382.

[53] Johnson LA, Aalbers JG, Willems CM, Sybesma W. Use of spermatozoa for artificial insemination. I. Fertilizing capacity of fresh and frozen spermatozoa in sows on 36 farms. J Anim Sci 1981;52: 1130-1136.

[54] Park CS, Yi YJ. Comparison of semen characteristics, sperm freezability and testosterone concentration between Duroc and Yorkshire boars during seasons. Anim Reprod Sci 2002;73: 53-61.

[55] Thurston LM, Siggins K, Mileham AJ, Watson PF, Holt WV. Identification of amplified restriction fragment length polymorphism markers linked to genes controlling boar sperm viability following cryopreservation. Biol Reprod 2002;66: 545-554.

[56] Pena FJ, Johannisson A, Wallgren M, Rodriguez Martinez H. Antioxidant supplementation in vitro improves boar sperm motility and mitochondrial membrane potential after cryopreservation of different fractions of the ejaculate. Anim Reprod Sci 2003;78: 85-98.

[57] Pena FJ, Saravia F, Nunez-Martinez I, Johannisson A, Wallgren M, Rodriguez Martinez H. Do different portions of the boar ejaculate vary in their ability to sustain cryopreservation? Anim Reprod Sci 2006;93: 101-113.

[58] Harrison RA, Ashworth PJ, Miller NG. Bicarbonate/CO2, an effector of capacitation, induces a rapid and reversible change in the lipid architecture of boar sperm plasma membranes. Mol Reprod Dev 1996;45: 378-391.

[59] Thurston LM, Watson PF, Mileham AJ, Holt WV. Morphologically distinct sperm subpopulations defined by Fourier shape descriptors in fresh ejaculates correlate with variation in boar semen quality following cryopreservation. J Androl 2001;22: 382-394.

[60] Zhu J, Xu X, Cosgrove JR, Foxeroft GR. Effects of semen plasma from different fractions of individual ejaculates on IVF in pigs. Theriogenology 2000;54: 1443-1452.

[61] Pursel VG, Johnson LA, Schulman LL. Effect of dilution, seminal plasma and incubation period on cold shock susceptibility of boar spermatozoa. J Anim Sci 1973;37: 528-531.

[62] Foulkes JA. The separation of lipoproteins from egg yolk and their effect on the motility and integrity of bovine spermatozoa. J Reprod Fertil 1977;49: 277-284.

[63] Gebauer MR, Pickett BW, Komarek RJ, Gaunya WS. Motility of bovine spermatozoa extended in "defined" diluents. J Dairy Sci 1970;53: 817-823.

[64] Wilmut I, Polge C. The low temperature preservation of boar spermatozoa. 1. The motility and morphology of boar spermatozoa frozen and thawed in the presence of permeating protective agents. Cryobiology 1977;14: 471-478.

[65] Wilmut I, Polge C. The low temperature preservation of boar spermatozoa. 2. The motility and morphology of boar spermatozoa frozen and thawed in diluent which contained only sugar and egg yolk. Cryobiology 1977;14: 479-482.

[66] Larsson K, Einarsson S, Swensson T. The development of a practicable method for deepfreezing of boar spermatozoa. Nord Vet Med 1977;29: 113-118.

[67] Bwanga CO. Cryopreservation of boar semen. I: A literature review. Acta Vet Scand 1991;32: 431-453.

[68] Fraser L, Strzezek J. Effect of different procedures of ejaculate collection, extenders and packages on DNA integrity of boar spermatozoa following freezing-thawing. Anim Reprod Sci 2007;99: 317-329.

[69] Pursel VG, Schulman LL, Johnson LA. Effect of Orvus ES Paste on acrosome morphology, motility and fertilizing capacity of frozen-thawed boar sperm. J Anim Sci 1978;47: 198-202.

[70] Axner E, Hermansson U, Linde-Forsberg C. The effect of Equex STM paste and sperm morphology on post-thaw survival of cat epididymal spermatozoa. Anim Reprod Sci 2004;84: 179-191.

[71] Eriksson BM, Rodriguez-Martinez H. Effect of freezing and thawing rates on the post-thaw viability of boar spermatozoa frozen in FlatPacks and Maxi-straws. Anim Reprod Sci 2000;63: 205-220.

[72] Pena AI, Lugilde LL, Barrio M, Herradon PG, Quintela LA. Effects of Equex from different sources on post-thaw survival, longevity and intracellular Ca2+ concentration of dog spermatozoa. Theriogenology 2003;59: 1725-1739.

[73] Arriola J, Foote RH. Glycerolation and thawing effects on bull spermatozoa frozen in detergent-treated egg yolk and whole egg extenders. J Dairy Sci 1987;70: 1664-1670.

[74] Penfold LM, Moore HD. A new method for cryopreservation of mouse spermatozoa. J Reprod Fertil 1993;99: 131-134.

[75] Eriksson BM, Rodriguez-Martinez H. Deep-freezing of boar semen in plastic film 'cochettes'. J Vet Med A Physiol Pathol Clin Med 2000;47: 89-97.

[76] Berger B, Fischerleitner F. On Deep Freezing of Boar Semen: Investigations on the Effects of Different Straw Volumes, Methods of Freezing and Thawing Extenders. Reproduction in Domestic Animals 1992;27: 266-270.

[77] Bwanga CO, de Braganca MM, Einarsson S, Rodriguez-Martinez H. Cryopreservation of Boar Semen in Mini- and Maxi-Straws. Journal of Veterinary Medicine Series A 1990;37: 651-658.

[78] Dube C, Beaulieu M, Reyes-Moreno C, Guillemette C, Bailey JL. Boar sperm storage capacity of BTS and Androhep Plus: viability, motility, capacitation, and tyrosine phosphorylation. Theriogenology 2004;62: 874-886.

[79] Vyt P, Maes D, Dejonckheere E, Castryck F, Van Soom A. Comparative study on five different commercial extenders for boar semen. Reprod Domest Anim 2004;39: 8-12.

[80] Nissen AK, Soede NM, Hyttel P, Schmidt M, D'Hoore L. The influence of time of insemination relative to time of ovulation on farrowing frequency and litter size in sows, as investigated by ultrasonography. Theriogenology 1997;47: 1571-1582.

[81] Curry MR. Cryopreservation of semen from domestic livestock. Rev Reprod 2000;5: 46-52.

[82] Eriksson BM, Petersson H, Rodriguez-Martinez H. Field fertility with exported boar semen frozen in the new flatpack container. Theriogenology 2002;58: 1065-1079.

[83] Watson PF, Behan JR. Intrauterine insemination of sows with reduced sperm numbers: results of a commercially based field trial. Theriogenology 2002;57: 1683-1693.

[84] Martinez EA, Vazquez JM, Roca J, Lucas X, Gil MA, Parrilla I, Vazquez JL, Day BN. Successful non-surgical deep intrauterine insemination with small numbers of spermatozoa in sows. Reproduction 2001;122: 289-296.

[85] Martinez EA, Vazquez JM, Roca J, Lucas X, Gil MA, Parrilla I, Vazquez JL, Day BN. Minimum number of spermatozoa required for normal fertility after deep intrauterine insemination in non-sedated sows. Reproduction 2002;123: 163-170.

[86] Roberts PK, Bilkei G. Field experiences on post-cervical artificial insemination in the sow. Reprod Domest Anim 2005;40: 489-491.

[87] Rozeboom KJ, Reicks DL, Wilson ME. The reproductive performance and factors affecting on-farm application of low-dose intrauterine deposit of semen in sows. J Anim Sci 2004;82: 2164-2168.

[88] Vazquez JM, Martinez EA, Parrilla I, Roca J, Gil MA, Vazquez JL. Birth of piglets after deep intrauterine insemination with flow cytometrically sorted boar spermatozoa. Theriogenology 2003;59: 1605-1614.

[89] Martinez EA, Caamano JN, Gil MA, Rieke A, McCauley TC, Cantley TC, Vazquez JM, Roca J, Vazquez JL, Didion BA, Murphy CN, Prather RS, Day BN. Successful nonsurgical deep uterine embryo transfer in pigs. Theriogenology 2004;61: 137-146.

[90] Martinez EA, Vazquez JM, Parrilla I, Cuello C, Gil MA, Rodriguez-Martinez H, Roca J, Vazquez JL. Incidence of unilateral fertilizations after low dose deep intrauterine insemination in spontaneously ovulating sows under field conditions. Reprod Domest Anim 2006;41: 41-47.

[91] Roca J, Carvajal G, Lucas X, Vazquez JM, Martinez EA. Fertility of weaned sows after deep intrauterine insemination with a reduced number of frozen-thawed spermatozoa. Theriogenology 2003;60: 77-87.

[92] Bolarin A, Roca J, Rodriguez-Martinez H, Hernandez M, Vazquez JM, Martinez EA. Dissimilarities in sows' ovarian status at the insemination time could explain differences in fertility between farms when frozen-thawed semen is used. Theriogenology 2006;65: 669-680.

[93] Wongtawan T, Saravia F, Wallgren M, Caballero I, Rodriguez-Martinez H. Fertility after deep intra-uterine artificial insemination of concentrated low-volume boar semen doses. Theriogenology 2006;65: 773-787.

[94] Buranaamnuay K, Tummaruk P, Singlor J, Rodriguez-Martinez H, Techakumphu M. Effects of straw volume and Equex-STM on boar sperm quality after cryopreservation. Reprod Domest Anim 2009;44: 69-73.

[95] Ponglowhapan S, Chatdarong K. Effects of Equex STM Paste on the quality of frozen-thawed epididymal dog spermatozoa. Theriogenology 2008;69: 666-672.

[96] Nothling JO, Shuttleworth R. The effect of straw size, freezing rate and thawing rate upon post-thaw quality of dog semen. Theriogenology 2005;63: 1469-1480.

[97] Buranaamnuay K, Singlor J, Tummaruk P, Techakumphu M. The establishment of boar semen cryopreservation in Thailand: post-thaw semen quality, sperm concentration and variation among ejaculates. Thai J Agri Sci 2008;41: 135-141.

[98] Larsson K, Einarsson S. Fertility of deep frozen boar spermatozoa: influence of thawing diluents and of boars. Acta Vet Scand 1976;17: 43-62.

[99] Buranaamnuay K, Y. P, Tummaruk P, Techakumphu M. Fertilization rate and number of embryos on day 2 after Intrauterine and deep intrauterine insemination using frozen-thawed boar semen in multiparous sows. Vet Med Inter 2011.

[100] Sumransap P, Tummaruk P, Kunavongkrit A. Sperm distribution in the reproductive tract of sows after intrauterine insemination. Reprod Domest Anim 2007;42: 113-117.

[101] Tummaruk P, Sumransap P, Techakumphu M, Kunavongkrit A. Distribution of spermatozoa and embryos in the female reproductive tract after unilateral deep intra uterine insemination in the pig. Reprod Domest Anim 2007;42: 603-609.

[102] Buranaamnuay K, Tummaruk P, Techakumphu M. Intra-uterine insemination with low numbers of frozen–thawed boar spermatozoa in spontaneous and induced ovulating sows under field conditions. Livestock Science 2010;131: 115-118.

[103] Bertani GR, Scheid IR, Fialho FB, Rubin MI, Wentz I, Goncalves PB. Effect of the time of artificial insemination with frozen-thawed or fresh semen on embryo viability and early pregnancy rate in gilts. Theriogenology 1997;48: 933-945.

[104] Waberski D, Weitze KF, Gleumes T, Schwarz M, Willmen T, Petzoldt R. Effect of time of insemination relative to ovulation on fertility with liquid and frozen boar semen. Theriogenology 1994;42: 831-840.

Chapter 3

The Use Of Sex-Sorted Sperm For Reproductive Programs In cattle

Gustavo Guerino Macedo,
Manoel Francisco de Sá Filho,
Rodrigo Vasconcelos Sala,
Márcio Ferreira Mendanha,
Evanil Pires de Campos Filho and
Pietro Sampaio Baruselli

Additional information is available at the end of the chapter

http://dx.doi.org/10.5772/52180

1. Introduction

The biotechnology of sex selection in animals is one of the most studied and also misunderstood in the history. According Garner and Seidel [1], Democratis (470 – 402 AC) had suggested that the right testicle produces male sperm and the left female. For sure that is not true, once there are two sperm populations on the mammals ejaculate, being a portion of it carrier the X sexual chromosome and other Y. During years, researchers have been trying to manipulate the sex of the offspring before conception [1]. The selection of desired sex delivered can be one of the determining factors to increase the genetic progress and farmer profitability in either beef or dairy cattle. For example, in dairy farms, the male calf has little or any zootechnical or economic value. However, in beef farms, the male calf is the product of interest due to its increased potential to produce meat. Considering these particularities, many researches have been developed to predict and/or manipulate the calf sex proportion. The separation of the Y sperm from the X is possible due to the differences on the DNA content of these spermatic cells (X sperm has about 4% more genetic material than Y) by flow cytometry. Nowadays, this is the most efficient method to separate X from Y-spermatozoa in large scale. Some available biotechnologies in commercial scale are the use of the sex-sorted sperm by artificial insemination (AI) with estrus detection, timed artificial insemination (TAI), embryo transfer with superovulation (ET) and timed embryo transfer (TET).

Reproductive programs based on TAI, have been continuously incorporated in routine of the reproductive management on farms. These programs represent a systematic approach to enhance the use of AI in dairy or beef farms, increasing the benefits of this reproductive biotechnology.

The ET technique has been used widely around the world once it increases the number of offspring that can be obtained from females with great genetic value [2, 3]. The use of sex-sorted sperm could increase the production of a specific calf gender, which would benefit beef and dairy industries worldwide [4]. Likewise, the TET synchronizes the ovulation similar to TAI; however, instead to inseminate before ovulation, the recipient cow receive an embryo fertilized *in vitro* with sex-sorted sperm seven days after ovulation.

Advances in sex sorting of sperm using flow cytometry have enabled its incorporation into commercial reproductive management. Despite the increased use of sex-sorted sperm, pregnancy per AI (P/AI) is still less than when using non sex-sorted sperm [5]. Regardless of these reduced results, suitable spermatozoa concentration at AI time; longer intervals from the induction of ovulation to the AI (i.e., closer to the expected moment of ovulation); AI into the uterine horn ipsilateral to the expected ovulation; the size of the follicle from which ovulation occurs; occurrence of estrus from progesterone (P4) source removal to the TAI and the identification and use of bulls with proven fertility producing spermatozoa resistant to the sexing process have increased the likelihood of pregnancy in females inseminated with sex-sorted sperm [6-8], thereby optimizing the use of sex-sorted sperm in TAI and ET programs.

There is a huge interest in sex-sorted sperm around the world. There are many opportunities and challenges associated to the use of this semen in farms. The aim of this review is to bring into focus a summary of our current understanding of the use of sex-sorted sperm in TAI and ET programs and some strategies to optimize the use of sex-sorted sperm. Before describing the researches results and opportunities for its use, it is important to understand how sperm are sorted and the critical points associated to the process.

2. Basic principles of sexing

The biotechnology of sex sorting is based on the information that X-sperm has about 4% more genetic material than Y-sperm. In this manner, the flow cytometry associates the laser, differential coloration of the viable and non-viable spermatozoa and hydrodynamic force which direct the sperm at the moment of the reading during the process of X and Y sperm separation. Moreover, there are differences among bovine breeds according to the amount of DNA present in the Y chromosome. According Garner [9], the X-Y sperm nuclei DNA content difference (%) is: 4.22 for Jersey, 4.07 for Angus, 4.01 for Holstein, 3.98 for Hereford and 3.7 for Brahman. Such differences, do not determine the fertility after sexing process. These differences mainly determine the speed and efficiency of the sexed semen production and have to be considered when using flow cytometry.

Recent advances in the form of the tip of the flow cytometry, the positioning of the sperm cells at the moment of the passage through the laser, as well as changes in pressure and the type of staining cells have significantly improved separation process gametes X and Y [9]. The X-Y sperm separation speed is relatively slow with approximately 300,000 to 400,000 cells per minute. In this way, for a higher process efficacy, the semen dose in the straw normally used is set to be 2.1 x 10^6 cells in a 0.25cc straw.

The process of sorting X and Y-bearing sperm likely results in some damage to the sperm that compromise fertilization [4, 10]. According to Gonsálvez et al. [11], the sorting process produce an interaction of the DNA with fluorophores, laser exposure, spermatozoa separation in micro-droplets, acceleration of spermatozoa through geometrically-pressured fluid channels and centrifugation. All of these para-biological spermatozoa-media or mechanical interactions would theoretically have the potential to produce changes in cell structures, including the DNA molecule. When considering cell structures, spermatozoa appear to be partially capacitated during the flow cytometry process used for sex pre-determination [12]. This total or partial capacitation is induced by the conditions that sperm are subjected during preparation for flow cytometric-sorting and during sorting [13]. Lu and Seidel [12] emphasize that it could be due to the condition that the sperm are pre-incubated with Hoechst 33342 at 34.5 8C for 45 min before sorting. During sorting, sperm are subjected to laser light and various physical forces, such as exiting the sorter at nearly 90 km/h before entering the collecting medium. The process of sorting results in an extremely diluted sample with 800,000 sperm/ml, and subsequently sperm are gently centrifuged to provide a concentrated sample suitable for packaging and cryopreservation.

Thus, this process could also led to a shorter functional sperm life compared to non-sorted sperm [12, 14, 15], which could include pre-capacitation and a reduced number of viable spermatozoa for the insemination [6, 16]. The thermo-resistance test showed that the motility decline in sex-sorted sperm was faster compared to non-sorted sperm. Also, there is an effect associated with samples from a specific bull and sex-sorted sperm insemination dose [5] and some samples from certain bulls can tolerate the stress of sorting in a more desirable manner [17].

Although the above information stated, it is important to highlight that AI with sex-sorted sperm does not alter pattern of return to estrus and does not affect the likelihood of heifers to conceive from subsequent AI [18]. Also, Holstein heifers inseminated with sexed semen had similar pregnancy loss from 29 ± 1 to 50 ± 1 d after AI compared with heifers inseminated with conventional semen [17], and there is no difference on abortion rate from 2 mo of gestation to parturition. Farmers in general are interested to know if calves produced by sexed semen are different that those from conventional semen. To address this question Tubman et al. [19] analyzed data from 1,169 calves produced from sexed semen and 793 calves from conventional semen. They did not observed difference in gestation length, birth weight, calving ease, calf vigor, weaning weight, abortion rate, and death rates (neonatal and through weaning) among calves produced by sexed or conventional semen. When *in vitro* models are used to verify the efficiency of sex-sorted sperm to produce embryos, there are inconsistent results concerning the embryo development which mainly depend on the sire used [20-22]. In general, P/AI of females inseminated with sex-sorted is not resultant from increased late embryonic and fetal losses. Therefore, calves produced from sexed semen grew and developed normally both pre- and postnatally.

3. Sperm concentration for sex-sorted sperm in reproductive programs

Commercially, the established spermatozoa number by dose of sexed semen is 2.1 x 10^6 cells/dose. This amount is much lower than that from conventional semen (~20 x 10^6 cells/dose). To achieve this proportion many studies have been done to specify the best straw concentration considering commercial aspects. Holstein heifers and cows have same conception rate when inseminated with sex-sorted sperm in a dose of 2.1 or 3.5 × 10^6 sperm/dose; however, not only in heifers but also in cows, there is an increasing on conception when AI is performed with conventionally processed sperm (15 x 10^6 sperm/dose) as presented on Table 1.

	Sex-sorted sperm (dose)		Non sex-sorted sperm (dose)
	2.1 x 10^6	3.5 x 10^6	15 × 10^6
Heifers (%)	43.9^a (2,752/6,268)	45.7^a (2,864/6,268)	60.7^b (3,805/6,268)
Cows (%)	23.0^a (1,257/5,466)	25,4^a (1,388/5,466)	31,5^b (1,722/5,466)

Table 1. Different superscript letters ($^{a, b}$) in row indicates statistical difference ($P < 0.01$).Adapted from Dejarnette et al. [23].Conception rates Holstein heifers and cows after artificial insemination with 2.1 or 3.5 × 10^6 sex-sorted sperm or 15 × 10^6 non sex-sorted sperm.

Dejarnette et al. [24] compared the effects of sperm dosage (2.1 vs. 10 × 10^6 sperm/dose) and sex-sorting (conventional vs. sexed) on conception rates of Holstein heifers (n = 9,172) and observed difference among groups as follows on Table 2. In a field trial study with three different breeds (Holstein, Jersey and Danish Red) Borchersen and Peacock [25] observed a reduction of 12% for Holstein, 7% for Jersey, and 5% for Danish Red in conception rate using sexed semen.

	Sperm dosage	
	2.1 x 10^6	10 x 10^6
Sex-sorted sperm (%)	38^a (881/2,319)	44^c (1,003/2,279)
Non sex-sorted sperm (%)	55^b (1,255/2,282)	60^d (1,375/2,292)

Table 2. Different superscript letters ($^{a, b, c}$ and ^{d}) indicates statistical difference ($P < 0.01$).Adapted from Dejarnette et al. [24].Conception rates of Holstein heifers according semen type (sexed vs. conventional) and sperm dosage combinations (2.1 vs. 10 × 10^6 sperm/dose).

In a combination of some experiments, Seidel et al. [26] observed that the conception rate of Holstein heifers inseminated with sex-sorted sperm vary from 40% to 68%, and with non-sex-sorted sperm vary from 67% to 82%. Also, Seidel and Schenk [17] observed a lower pregnancy rate when using sex-sorted sperm (31% to 42%) than non sex-sorted sperm (43% to 62%). Although the greater variability on the pregnancy outcomes of cattle inseminated of with sex-sorted sperm by literature, most part of the researches with heifers indicates that conception rate after AI upon estrous detection with sex-sorted sperm is about 70% to 90% (according to the farms handling) from the conception obtained following the use of conventional semen [27]. In accordance, Sá Filho et al. [28] showed that overall P/AI rates were reduced with sex-sorted sperm compared with non sex-sorted sperm (i.e., 83.8% pregnancy was obtained with the non-sex-sorted sperm). This reduced P/AI could be attributable to several factors including a shorter lifespan in the female reproductive tract, reduced number of sperm per straw, and sperm damage from the staining, identification, and separation processes [5, 6, 14]. The Table 3 summarizes the main studies with sex-sorted sperm, stating the pregnancy rate and the proportion of pregnancy sexed/conventional semen.

In a first report to evaluate the fertility of lactating dairy cows under field conditions, females where inseminated with same low concentration (2×10^6) of sex-sorted or non sex-sorted frozen-thawed sperm [29], it was observed the same pregnancy per AI among females inseminated with sex-sorted (27.6%, n = 105) or non sex-sorted (28.1%, n = 64) sperm. Although the inconsistent results with cows presented by literature, most part of the researches with heifers indicates that conception rate after estrus detection by observation and AI with sex-sorted sperm is about 70% to 90% (it depends on to the farms handling) form the conception rate obtained by conventional semen [27].

Considering that maybe straw concentration would still be low, our research group performed an experiment inseminating Jersey heifers once or twice [7]. Aimed at, 576 virgin Jersey heifers were synchronized with two injections of PGF2α apart and had their estrus observed twice daily (based upon removal of tail-head chalk). The AI was performed with a single insemination dose (2.1×10^6 sperm) 12 h after estrus detection (n=193), a double dose at 12 h (n=193), or a double dose involving insemination 12 and 24 h after estrus detection (n=190). It was not observed any effect of treatments on P/AI (87/193 = 45.1%, 85/193 = 44.0%, and 94/190 = 49.5%, respectively; P = 0.51). However, P/AI was influenced by the number of AI service (First, 115/208 = 55.3%[a]; Second, 94/204 = 46.1%[a]; and Third, 57/165 = 34.8%[b]; P = 0.004). Similar results have also been described by Dejarnette et al. [30] where, pregnancy rate has been reduced in heifers when the number of AI service has been increased (First service = 47%; Second = 39% ; Third = 32%). Accordingly, in Jersey heifers, the increasing on the spermatozoa number, 2.1 to 4.2 million, to be used in insemination after estrus detection and to perform a double insemination (12 hour interval) have not changed the conception rate.

The use of sex-sorted sperm in suckled beef cows in the post-partum have not been much explored scientifically. Most part of the papers use few cows per treatment, making the results inconclusive. A study in suckled Angus cows (n = 212), Doyle et al. [34] compared the following treatments:

1. Frozen conventional semen (40 x 10^6 sperm/dose) deposited at uterus corpus;
2. Frozen conventional semen at low concentration (1 x 10^6 sperm/dose);
3. Frozen sexed semen (1 x 10^6 sperm/dose);
4. Cooled sexed semen (5 x 10^6 sperm/dose).

Semen for the Treatment 1 was deposited into the uterus corpus. Semen for the other three treatments was shared where each half was deposited into each uterine horn. Pregnancy was lower for the sex-sorted sperm treatments (frozen = 23% and cooled = 25%) than for the non sex-sorted sperm (conventional = 67% and low concentration = 49%)

		Pregnancy rate based on type of semen used in AI			
Breed	Category	Conventional (%) (n/n)	Sexed (%) (n/n)	Proportion (%)	Reference
Timed Artificial insemination					
Beef	Cows	54.2 (232/428)	45.4 (193/425)	83.7	Sá Filho et al. [31] (Exp 1)
Beef	Cows	54.7 (134/245)	45.9 (113/246)	83.9	Sá Filho et al. [31] (Exp 2)
Beef	Cows	51.8 (100/193)	41.8 (82/196)	80.7	Sales et al. [8]
Beef	Cows	55.3 (105/190)	40.9 (79/193)	74.0	Sales et al. [8]
Dairy	Cows	27.1 (44/162)	13.0 (21/161)	48.0	Souza et al. 2006 unpublished data
Artificial insemination with estrus detection					
Beef	Heifers	67.6 (96/142)	53.7 (130/242)	79.4	Seidel and Schenk [17] (Exp.1)
Beef	Heifers	67.0 (85/126)	52.6 (129/245)	78.5	Seidel and Schenk [17] (Exp.2)
Dairy	Heifers	60.0 (1375/2292)	38.0 (881/2319)	63.3	DeJarnette et al. [24]
Dairy	Cows and Heifers	37.7 (160/426)	22.9 (51/223)	60.7	Mellado et al. [32]
Dairy	Heifers	56.0 (30082/53718)	45.0 (17893/39763)	80.3	DeJarnette et al. [30]
Dairy	Cows and Heifers	37.4 (34/91)	28.8 (38/132)	77.0	Bodmer et al. [29]
Dairy	Cows	46.0 (69/149)	21.0 (33/157)	45.6	Andersson et al. [33]

		Pregnancy rate based on type of semen used in AI			
Dairy	Heifers	60.0 (74/124)	46.7 (114/244)	77.8	Seidel and Schenk [17] (Exp.4)
Dairy	Heifers	62.0 (163/263)	42.1 (225/534)	67.9	Seidel and Schenk [17] (Exp.5)
Overall		55.9% (32753/58549)	44.3% (19982/45080)	79.2	

Table 3. Pregnancy rate of females inseminated with conventional or sexed semen and the pregnancy proportion obtained by sexed semen based on conventional. (sexed/conventional).

In brief, the fertility of cows and heifers is influenced when the dose of the sex-sorted sperm is considerably increased [for example to 10 x 10^6 sperm/AI; [24]]. However, the high cost of increasing the insemination dose would make this commercially unviable. Certainly duo to the low sorting rate per hour provided by flow cytometry method. Nowadays, sexing companies just offer sexed semen in a dose of 2.1 x 10^6 sperm/straw, and studies have been done using this dose as pattern'. Also, data suggest a better use of sex-sorted sperm in the first/second service.

4. Timing for AI using non sex-sorted or sex-sorted sperm

4.1. AI following estrus detection

The optimal time at which insemination should take place relative to ovulation (IOI) depends primarily on the lifespan of spermatozoa and on the viability of the oocyte in the female genital tract [35]. Several experiments [36-38] have demonstrated that 6 h is the minimum time needed for a viable sperm population capable of fertilization to pass through the oviduct. Furthermore, the number of progressive motile sperm peaked from 8 to 18 h after insemination. In terms of the oocyte, the most desirable period for fertilization appears to be between 6 and 10 h after ovulation [39]. Also, Dransfield et al. [40] and Roelofs et al. [41] demonstrated that the probability that conception will occur decreases when AI is performed near the time of ovulation (less than 12 or 6 h before ovulation, respectively). According to Roelofs et al. [42], fertilization rate drastically decreases when AI occurs after ovulation. Artificial insemination should occur near the time of ovulation to maximize sperm access to the ovum, but not so late that an aging ovum awaits sperm arrival [43]. The ovulation occurs 28-30 h after the estrus beginning. The optimal AI time was between 24 and 12 h before ovulation for the most desirable rate of fertilization and 16–12 h for greatest percentage of greater quality embryos [89% of recovered embryos; [42]. More precisely, Maatje et al. [44] obtained an optimal pregnancy rate when AI was performed 16.2 h before ovulation.

In a review by Seidel et al. [26], crossbred beef heifers inseminated with sex-sorted sperm, present conception rate about 40%, lower than AI with non sex-sorted sperm (75%).

Sá Filho et al. [7] have been evaluated the different times to perform the AI. Thereby, 638 Jersey heifers have been inseminated after estrus detection according those times (12 a 16h; 16 a 20h; 20 a 24h e 24 a 30h) and the estrus has been detected using radio telemetry (Heat Watch®). The P/AI of heifers inseminated from 12 to 16 h after the onset of estrus ($40/10^6$ = 37.7%) was less (P = 0.03) than those inseminated from 16.1 to 20 h (85/164 = 51.8%), and 20.1 to 24 h (130/234 = 55.6%). However, the P/AI for heifers inseminated from 24.1 to 30 h (61/134 = 45.5%) did not differ from that of any other interval.

Pharmacological manipulation is expected to increase the reproductive performance even in management with estrus detection. Exogenous GnRH given at the onset of estrus [45, 46] or concurrent with AI [47, 48] have improved fertility, but the effects have not been consistent [45-48]. Therefore, reproductive strategies to enhance fertility with exogenous hormones, optimizing estrus detection, or improving the timing of AI relative to estrus detection, could enhance the use of sexed semen in dairy cattle breeding. Following this idea, our group aimed to develop strategies to improve P/AI (35 to 42 d after AI) in virgin Jersey heifers bred by AI of sex-sorted sperm after being detected in estrus [7]. Nevertheless, giving 100 μg of GnRH at first detection of estrus, with AI 12 h later, did not affect P/AI in females with estrus detected by tail-head chalk [GnRH=47.2% (100/212) vs. No GnRH=51.7% (104/201); P = 0.38] or by radio telemetry [HeatWatch® ; GnRH=53.1% (137/258) vs. No GnRH=48.6% (122/251); P = 0.43]. In the referred study, GnRH treatments were done 7.4 h after the onset of estrus, identified by HeatWatch® system, due to the management schedule (i.e. twice daily 07:00 or 19:00). Previous studies demonstrated that the onset of estrus, the peak of the 17β-estradiol in plasma, and the release of the ovulatory LH surge occurred at approximately the same moment [49, 50]. However, treatment with GnRH following a spontaneous LH surge resulted in a surge of LH of shorter duration and decreased magnitude compared to an ovulatory LH surge [51]. Additionally, treatment with GnRH at AI tended to decrease subsequent progesterone concentrations in synchronized beef heifers [48]. Therefore, the positive effect of GnRH treatment at estrus appeared to be most beneficial in females with decreased fertility, or when the treatment was performed close to the onset of estrus (i.e., close to the spontaneous LH surge).

4.2. AI following synchronization of ovulation

The use of a P4/progestin plus E2 based TAI protocols has been the most commercially used type of fixed time synchronization protocol in South America [52-55]. In females, a common aspect among the estrus synchronization protocols for TAI is the insertion of an intravaginal device containing P4 or an ear implant containing norgestomet plus administration of estradiol benzoate (EB; 2mg i.m.) on Day 0; an injection of prostaglandin (PG) F2α on Day 8 or 9 at the moment of device withdrawal plus 300 to 400 IU of equine chorionic gonadotropin (eCG). Different ovulation inducers with similar efficiency could be used such as estradiol cipionate (EC; 0.5 mg i.m.) at moment or EB (1mg i.m.) 24 h after the P4/progestin implant removal. Timed artificial insemination use to occur 48 to 60 hours after P4/progestin source withdrawal [54-58].

A possibility to improve the use of sex-sorted sperm is controlling the ovulation time variation through the use of synchronization techniques; thus, increasing the efficiency of AI programs using sexed semen. For instance, in beef and dairy cows, P4 and E2 based synchronization induce ovulation around 70-72h after the P4 device removal [59-61].

The P4-based synchronization protocol is a well-established protocol to synchronize the ovulation. Despite the satisfactory predictability of the moment of ovulation provided by the P4 plus estradiol-based estrus synchronization protocol (averaging 66 to 72 h after P4 device removal), the timing of ovulation is influenced by the diameter of the follicle at the time of the ovulatory stimulus treatment [62]. Neves [62] evaluated the time of ovulation in a large number of suckled *Bos indicus* cows (n = 312) and observed a significant effect of the diameter of the ovulatory follicle at the moment of synchronized ovulation (average of 71.8 ± 7.7 h after P4 device removal). The author reported that cows experiencing premature ovulation (i.e., ovulation occurring from 48 to 59 h after P4 device removal) presented a larger ovulatory follicle (14.0 ± 2.2 mm) than cows with delayed ovulation (11.4 ± 2.2 mm; 73 to 96 h after P4 device removal) and that cows that ovulated at the expected time of ovulation (60 to 72 h after P4 device removal) showed ovulatory follicles of intermediate diameter (13.6 ± 2.1 mm).

Once the sex-sorted sperm present lower viability on the reproductive tract than conventional semen [6, 14], our research group has evaluated the delay on AI using of sex-sorted sperm in heifers. A study [8] breeding 420 cyclic Jersey heifers at either 54 or 60 h after P4-device removal, using either sex-sorted (2.1 x 10^6 sperm/straw) or non-sorted sperm (20 x 10^6 sperm/straw) from three sires (2 x 2 factorial design). There was an interaction ($P = 0.06$) between time of AI and type of semen on pregnancy per AI (P/AI, at 30 to 42 d after TAI); it was greater when sex-sorted sperm ($P < 0.01$) was used at 60 h (31.4%; 32/102) than at 54 h (16.2%; 17/105). In contrast, altering the timing of AI did not affect conception results with non-sorted sperm (54 h = 50.5%; 51/101 versus 60 h = 51.8%; 58/112; $P = 0.95$). There was an effect of sire ($P < 0.01$) on P/AI, but no interaction between sire and time of AI ($P = 0.88$).

Based on previous results, Sales et al. [8] evaluated the ideal period to perform the TAI with sex-sorted sperm in a P4-based protocol of synchronization of ovulation. Suckled *Bos indicus* cows (n = 339) were randomly assigned to receive TAI with sex-sorted sperm at 36, 48, or 60 h after P4 device removal. Ultrasonographic examinations were performed twice daily in all cows to confirm ovulation. On average, ovulation occurred 71.8 ± 7.8 h after P4 removal, and greater P/AI was achieved when insemination was performed closer to ovulation. The P/AI was greatest (37.9%, 36/95) for TAI performed between 0 and 12 h before ovulation, whereas P/AI was significantly less for TAI performed between 12.1 and 24 h (19.4%, 21/108) or > 24 h (5.8%, 5/87) before ovulation ($P = 0.001$) as shown on Table 4. In the Table 5, it is presented a summary of studies when AI with sex-sorted sperm is performed at different times after protocol of synchronization of ovulation.

Interval from TAI to ovulation (h)	No. cows	Pregnant (%) No./No.	Adjusted OR[x] (95% CI)	P
"/ 24	87	5.8 (5/87)[c]	0.24 (0.08-0.70)	0.01
"/ 12 to 24	108	19.4 (21/108)[b]	Reference group	
"/ 0 to 12	95	37.9 (36/95)[a]	2.34 (1.22-4.51)	0.01
After ovulation[z]	22	36.4 (8/22)[ab]	1.80 (0.64-5.03)	0.27

Table 4. a,b Within a column, proportions without a common superscript differed (P _ 0.05).x OR, odds ratio; CI, confidence interval.y Reference, reference group for adjusted risk ratio, which is the industry standard for the optimal timing of AI with non-sorted sperm.z Inseminations were performed within 0–12 h after ovulation.Adapted from [8]Risk of pregnancy based on the interval between TAI and ovulation in suckled B. indicus cows inseminated with sex-sorted sperm.

		Pregnancy per AI % (n/n)		
Reference	Animal category	Early AI time	Late AI time	P *value*
Sales et al. (2011) [8]	Suckled Nelore cows	42.8 (100/193)	50.8 (99/195)	0.11
Schenk et al. (2009) [6]	Angus heifers	34 (11/32)	49 (17/35)	"/0.10
Sales et al. (2010) [63]	Jersey heifers	16.2 (17/105)	31.4 (32/102)	<0.05
Neves et al. (2010) [62]	Nelore cows	20.8 (27/130)	30.9 (38/123)	<0.05
Overall		25.1 (92/366)	37.0 (123/357)	<0.01

Table 5. Influence of the AI moment in synchronization of ovulation protocols on the pregnancy rate.

Importantly to note, the use of in vitro fertilized (IVF) embryos with sexed semen is expected to have its use increased throughout the years associated to TET. The overall percentages of oocytes fertilized with sorted and unsorted frozen bovine sperm appear to be similar using current IVF methods [20]. While TAI uses one dose of sexed semen by cow, the TET allows the optimization of the semen use. Just one sexed semen dose is capable to fertilize about 80 oocytes (equivalent to the aspiration of four females; mean of 20 oocytes per aspirated cow), resulting in the production of approximately 30 viable embryos. Considering that TET provides 40 – 50% of pregnancy rate, transferring the 30 embryos fertilized with just one sexed semen dose, would result theoretically, in 12 – 15 pregnancies. In the case where for TAI is considered the same conception rate of 40 – 50%, each inseminated sexed semen dose would result in just 0.4 – 0.5 pregnancies.

http://dx.doi.org/10.5772/52180

5. Bull effect on the efficiency of reproductive programs using sex-sorted sperm

An important factor to consider in the timing of AI with sex-sorted sperm is the variation in the fertility of individual bulls. Whereas sperm sorting has significantly decreased fertility of certain bulls, sperm sorting does not affect fertility of other bulls [25]. Sales et al. [63] have been evaluated the use of the sexed or conventional semen of 3 different sires to inseminate Jersey heifers after the estrus detection by radio telemetry (Heat Watch®). Wherefore, the conventional semen [64.2% (238/371)] had been a higher conception rate than sexed semen [49.5% (189/382); P = 0.001]. Moreover, there was a bull effect on the conception rate [Bull A = 50.0% (108/216)b; Bull B = 63.4% (211/333)a and Bull C = 53.5% (107/200)b; P = 0.008]. Thus, some bulls can present lower conception rate using sexed or conventional semen for insemination (Figure 1). Other studies also have described that conception rates vary in magnitude for individual sires [5, 25, 64].

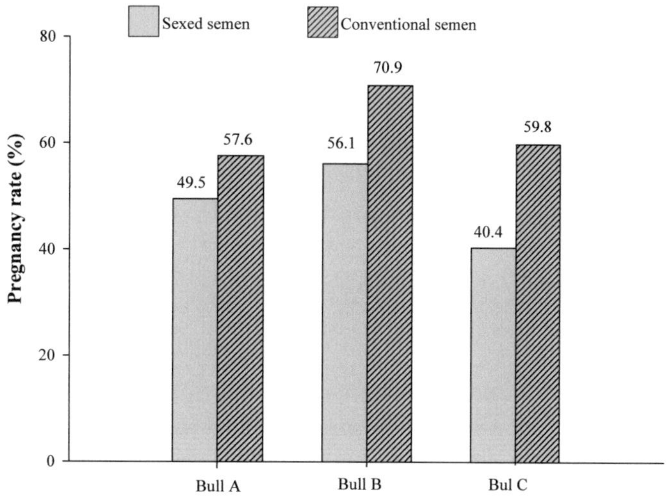

Figure 1. Conception rate of Jersey heifers inseminated artificially with sexed or conventional semen according three different the bull (A, n=216; B, n= 333 e C, n=200). Bull effect (P = 0.008) and semen (P = 0.001).

In another study, Sales et al. [8] synchronized Jersey heifers and used sex-sorted sperm from three different sires to inseminate the females. The conception rate was different among sires used in the experiment, indicating once more the existence of individual discrepancy among bulls producing semen to sex-sorting (Figure 2).

The few number of sorting facilities around the world limits the use of high genetic merit bulls because the distance. The capacity to effectively sex-sort and re-freeze previously frozen-thawed sperm would allow commercial sorting undertaking to offer sex-sorted sperm from any sire currently in the frozen semen market. This capacity is mainly influenced by variation in the physic-chemical semen properties of the individual bull. A study [65] to verify the fertilizing potential of sex-sorted frozen-thawed bull sperm transported cooled or frozen to the sorting facility, has shown a bull effect on the pregnancy rate after AI [Bull 1: conventional semen (control) 63.0%; previously frozen (FS) 8.6%; previously cooled (CS) 10.0%. Bull 2: control 45.5%, FS 0%, CS 4.8%; P = 0.001].

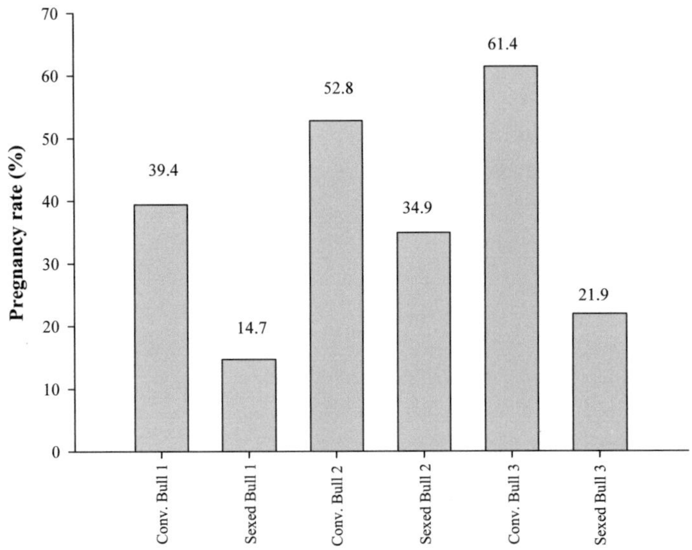

Figure 2. Pregnancy rate of Jersey heifers fixed timed artificially inseminated according the bull and type of semen used (conventional or sexed). It was verified a bull effect (P = 0.001) and type of semen (P = 0.001).

Accordingly, the individual difference among bull is an important aspect to consider applying the sex-sorted sperm use at livestock level, allowing the sire selection for higher performance after sexing. Also, it is essential to highlight that this sire effect is one of the most important obstacle to the use of sexed semen in large scale.

6. Use of sex-sorted sperm in superovulation protocol for embryo production

The use of sex sorted sperm in reproduction program using superovulation to produce female calf in dairy farms or male in beef farms have been used progressively. Our research group has studied this aspect in Nelore (*Bos indicus*) cows superovulated and inseminated with sex-sorted sperm. Animals were synchronized at Day 0 with norgestomet ear implant (Crestar®, MSD) with 2 mg of estradiol benzoate i.m. (Sincrodiol®, Ourofino). The follicle super stimulation was done was induced with 8 decreasing doses of pFSH (12/12 h) beginning on Day 4). On Day 6, was given PGF2α analog (Sincrocio®, Ourofino). The ear implant was removed 36 h after the PGF2α analog administration, with the application of LH (Luteotropin) 48 h after PGF2α analog. The TAI with sex-sorted (4,2x10^6 cell/AI) or non sex-sorted sperm (40x10^6 cell/AI) was performed at 12 and 24 h after LH injection. For TAI, it was used semen from same sire. The experimental design used was crossover to avoid individual variation among donors. The Table 6 summarizes the experiment described, demonstrating a decreasing on fresh and frozen embryos, fresh and frozen embryo rate and an increasing on the unfertilized embryos when using sex-sorted sperm. The accuracy on the use of the sexed semen to produce the desired sex was 90% with pregnancy diagnosis 60 days after TAI. The conventional semen produced 52.7% of females.

	Non sex-sorted sperm (n = 10)	**Sex-sorted sperm (n = 10)**	**Trat**	**Rep**	**Trat vs. Rep**
Total of structures (n)	9.90 ± 0.78	8.40 ± 1.40	0.28	0.81	0.71
Transferable embryos (Grade 1, 2 and 3; n)	6.80 ± 0.66	4.20 ± 0.74	0.03	0.88	0.88
Frozen embryos (Grade 1 and 2; n)	5.9 ± 0.71	3.50 ± 0.65	0.03	0.43	0.99
Unfertilized oocyte (n)	1.50 ± 0.48	3.70 ± 0.88	0.01	0.82	0.46
Degenerate (n)	1.60 ± 0.37	0.50 ± 0.16	0.04	0.54	0.78
Transferable embryo rate (%)	68.70 ± 6.30	50.00 ± 5.10	0.01	0.68	0.54
Frozen embryo rate (%)	59.60 ± 5.10	41.70 ± 5.20	0.02	0.32	0.73

Table 6. Embryo production of superovulated Nelore cows (*Bos indicus*) and inseminated in fixed time with sex-sorted or non sex-sorted sperm.

In a study by our group research [66], we evaluated different intervals for TAI with sex-sorted sperm after pLH treatment in *Bos indicus* and *Bos taurus* donors. The hypothesis was that increased embryo production would occur when TAI with sex-sorted sperm was performed closer to the time synchronized ovulations occurred. In the first experiment, hormonal superstimulation of ovarian follicular development in Nelore donors (n = 71) was performed in randomly allocated animals to one of three treatment groups, and they were inseminated at 12 and 24 h after an ovulatory stimulus with pLH treatment was applied, either with sex-sorted (4.2 x 10^6 sperm/insemination; S12/24; n = 17) or non-sorted sperm (20 x 10^6 sperm/insemination; NS12/24; n = 18), or they were inseminated at 18 and 30 h using sex-sorted sperm (4.2 x 10^6 sperm/insemination; S18/30; n = 19). A greater number of transferable embryos were found when sex-sorted sperm was used to inseminate the animals at 18 and 30 h compared to insemination at 12 and 24 h. However, a greater embryo production was obtained with non-sorted sperm (results are summarized on Table 7).

Additionally, Soares et al. [66] used the same insemination times and semen types in lactating high-production Holstein cows (n = 12). A crossover design was employed in this trial.

A lesser embryo production (0.007) was found in Holstein donors that were inseminated using sex-sorted sperm at 12 and 24 h compared to non-sorted sperm. However, intermediate results were obtained when the inseminations with sex-sorted sperm were performed at 18 and 30 h (Table 8).

	Treatments			**P value**
	Conventional 12/24	Sexed 12/24	Sexed 18/30	
Number of cows	17	18	19	----
Total ova/embryos	8.0 ± 3.2	7.1 ± 3.3	9.0 ± 3.8	0.14
Transferable embryos (n)	6.8 ± 2.6^{a}	2.4 ± 1.8^{c}	4.5 ± 3.0^{b}	< 0.001
Transferable embryos (%)^{d}	86.1 ± 11.9^{a}	37.3 ± 26.7^{c}	48.2 ± 25.9^{b}	< 0.001
Freezable embryos (n)	6.0 ± 2.4^{a}	2.0 ± 1.4^{c}	3.7 ± 2.8^{b}	< 0.001
Freezable embryos (%)^{e}	76.3 ± 19.2^{a}	31.8 ± 24.5^{c}	38.0 ± 26.5^{b}	< 0.001
Degenerate embryos	0.7 ± 0.7	0.9 ± 1.6	1.6 ± 2.1	0.05
Unfertilized oocytes	0.5 ± 0.7^{a}	3.7 ± 3.6^{b}	2.9 ± 2.6^{b}	< 0.001

Table 7. Rows with different superscripts (a, b, e) indicate P < 0.05. ^{d} Percentage of transferable embryos based on the number of ova/embryos recovered. ^{e} Percentage of freezable embryos based on the number of ova/embryos recovered.Adapted from Soares et al. [66].Embryo production of Nelore cows (*Bos indicus*) superovulated and inseminated in different times with conventional or sexed semen.

	Treatments			P *value*
	Conventional 12/24	Sexed 12/24	Sexed 18/30	
Number of cows	11	11	11	----
Total ova/embryos	10.4 ± 3.4	11.3 ± 4.4	12.4 ± 3.8	0.40
Transferable embryos (n)	8.7 ± 2.8^{a}	4.6 ± 3.0^{b}	6.4 ± 3.1^{ab}	0.007
Transferable embryos (%)^{d}	85.9 ± 14.0^{a}	40.7 ± 21.3^{c}	54.2 ± 23.2^{b}	< 0.001
Freezable embryos (n)	6.9 ± 1.8^{a}	3.2 ± 1.8^{b}	5.4 ± 3.4^{ab}	0.007
Freezable embryos (%)^{e}	69.9 ± 16.8^{a}	29.9 ± 15.5^{c}	45.3 ± 26.6^{b}	< 0.001
Degenerate embryos	0.7 ± 0.9	1.4 ± 1.8	1.3 ± 1.7	0.43
Unfertilized oocytes	0.9 ± 1.4^{a}	5.2 ± 3.1^{b}	4.6 ± 2.6^{b}	0.0003

Table 8. Rows with different superscripts (a, b, c) indicate P < 0.05. ^{d} Percentage of transferable embryos based on the number of ova/embryos recovered. ^{e} Percentage of freezable embryos based on the number of ova/embryos recovered.Adapted from Soares et al. [66].Embryo production of Holstein cows (*Bos Taurus*) superovulated and inseminated in different times with conventional or sexed semen.

Briefly, it is possible to improve embryo production using sex-sorted sperm in *Bos indicus* and *Bos taurus* superstimulated donors when the inseminations are performed near the same time as time-synchronized ovulations. However, the embryo production for TAI with sex-sorted sperm was still less than the production with non-sorted sperm.

7. Strategies to increase the pregnancy in TAI with sex-sorted sperm

After determining the best moment to perform the TAI with sex-sorted sperm, some studies were conducted aiming to verify the effect estrus expression and follicle diameter at the moment of TAI on the conception rate. Earlier studies have demonstrated that females displaying estrus before TAI have better ovarian responses [67] and with bigger follicle size at the moment of TAI [68] have better conception rate when AI is performed with conventional semen. When using this method of the follicle size on TAI with sex-sorted sperm [31], there is an interaction (P = 0.02) between the type of semen and the size of the dominant follicle [conventional ≥ 8mm = 58.9% (126/214); conventional < 8mm = 49.5% (101/204); sexed semen ≥ 8mm = 56.8% (134/236) and sexed semen < 8mm = 31.2% (59/189)]. In this study, it was verified that the difference between the type of semen used (conventional vs. sexed) on the pregnancy probability at 30 days, decrease according the dominant follicle size increase at TAI (P = 0.001).

There is an influence of the number of services with sex sorted sperm and the conception rate in heifers. It was observed by Sá filho et al. [7] working with Jersey heifers (n = 573) showed that P/AI was influenced by the number of AI service (First, 115/208 = 55.3%a; Second, 94/204 = 46.1%a; and Third, 57/165 = 34.8%b; P = 0.004). Similar results were achieved in a study by Dejarnette et al. [30] where pregnancy rate reduced in heifers with more AI service (First = 47%, Second = 39%, and Third = 32%). Thus, heifers which use to fail in the first AI probably will have their pregnancy rate compromised in the later services.

Vazquez et al. [69] in an interesting review, states that the sex-sorted spermatozoa are 'weakened' by the process, giving them a short functional lifespan. Consequently, new AI strategies are necessary in order to achieve high pregnancy rates with a low dose of sex-sorted spermatozoa. The deposition of the spermatozoa higher in the reproductive tract, compared with conventional AI, allows a greater proportion of spermatozoa to survive and colonize the oviduct. Therefore, fewer spermatozoa are necessary to achieve the same probability of fertility than with a dose deposited in a lower part of the reproductive tract, especially when weak spermatozoa are inseminated. However, in a recent study, Sá Filho et al. [31] compared the conception rate of a total of 200 suckled cows presenting LF ≥ 9 mm at TAI were randomly assigned to receive sex-sorted sperm deposited into the uterine body (n = 100) or into the uterine horn ipsilateral to the recorded LF (n = 100). No effect of deeper artificial insemination on P/AI was found (P = 0.57). Several studies have been performed to evaluate the effect of uterine horn insemination [70-77]. The majority of those previous results support the idea that site of semen deposition would play little to no role in P/AI. However, due to the presumably reduced viability of sexed sperm, the insemination closer to the site of ovulation would potentially provide better results [64, 78]. Also, it is important to mention that in most of those studies, the cornual inseminations were performed by depositing half of the semen straw into the right horn and the other half into the left horn. In the Sá Filho et al. [31] study, the insemination was performed with the full dose in the uterine horn ipsilateral to the expected side of ovulation. Despite these differences, similar P/AI was found when comparing inseminations performed in the horn or in the body of the uterus, which agrees with those previous results with conventional semen.

8. Conclusion

The sex sorting process by flow cytometry is aggressive to the spermatozoa, compromising the viability of these cells. Thus, some adjustments in the mode of use the sexed semen in AI have to be done to improve the tangibility in reproductive programs at livestock level. Adjustments in the AI moment in relation to the estrus beginning improve the conception rate. The results of the studies presented, indicates that beef and dairy heifers inseminated with sex-sorted sperm after estrus detection have satisfactory conception rate, and the AI has to be done between 16 to 24 h after the estrus commencement (6 to 14 h before ovulation). Also, when using synchronization of ovulation protocols for TAI in beef and dairy cows, acceptable conception rate is obtained when TAI is done at 60 h after P4 device removal (10 h before ovulation). Additionally, there is a huge individual variation of fertility among semen of sires submitted to the sexing process, and has to be considered at the moment of bull choosing in AI programs.

Author details

Gustavo Guerino Macedo[1], Manoel Francisco de Sá Filho[1], Rodrigo Vasconcelos Sala[1], Márcio Ferreira Mendanha[1], Evanil Pires de Campos Filho[2] and Pietro Sampaio Baruselli[1]

1 Departamento de Reprodução Animal, Faculdade de Medicina Veterinária e Zootecnia, Universidade de São Paulo, Brasil

2 Sexing Technologies, Sertãozinho, Brasil

References

[1] Gardner, D., & Seidel, G. (2008). History of commercializing sexed semen for cattle. *Theriogenology*, 69, 886-95.

[2] Baruselli, P. S., de Sá Filho, M. F., Martins, C. M., Nasser, L. F., Nogueira, M. F. G., Barros, C. M., et al. (2006). Superovulation and embryo transfer in Bos indicus cattle. *Theriogenology*, 65(1), 77-88.

[3] Bó, G. A., Baruselli, P. S., Chesta, P. M., & Martins, C. M. (2006). The timing of ovulation and insemination schedules in superstimulated cattle. *Theriogenology*, 65(1), 89-101.

[4] Sartori, R., Souza, A. H., Guenther, J. N., Caraviello, D. Z., Geiger, L. N., Schenk, J. L., et al. (2004). Fertilization rate and embryo quality in superovulated Holstein heifers artificially inseminated with X-sorted or unsorted sperm. *Animal Reproduction*, 1, 86-90.

[5] De Jarnette, J. M., Nebel, R. L., Marshall, C. E., Moreno, J. F., Mc Cleary, C. R., & Lenz, R. W. (2008). Effect of Sex-Sorted Sperm Dosage on Conception Rates in Holstein Heifers and Lactating Cows. *Journal of dairy science*, 91(5), 1778-85.

[6] Schenk, J. L., Cran, D. G., Everett, R. W., & Seidel, G. E. (2009). Pregnancy rates in heifers and cows with cryopreserved sexed sperm: Effects of sperm numbers per inseminate, sorting pressure and sperm storage before sorting. *Theriogenology*, 71(5), 717-28.

[7] Sá Filho, M. F., Ayres, H., Ferreira, R. M., Nichi, M., Fosado, M., Campos, Filho. E. P., et al. (2010). Strategies to improve pregnancy per insemination using sex-sorted semen in dairy heifers detected in estrus. *Theriogenology*, 74(9), 1636-42.

[8] Sales, J. N. S., Neves, K. A. L., Souza, A. H., Crepaldi, G. A., Sala, R. V., Fosado, M., et al. (2011). Timing of insemination and fertility in dairy and beef cattle receiving timed artificial insemination using sex-sorted sperm. *Theriogenology*, 76(3), 427-35.

[9] Garner, D. L. (2006). Flow cytometric sexing of mammalian sperm. *Theriogenology*, 65(5), 943-57.

[10] Garner, G. E. S. D. (2002). Current status of sexing mammalian spermatozoa. *Reproduction*, 124(6), 733-43.

[11] Gosálvez, J., Ramirez, M. A., López-Fernández, C., Crespo, F., Evans, K. M., Kjelland, M. E., et al. (2011). Sex-sorted bovine spermatozoa and DNA damage: I. *Static features. Theriogenology*, 75(2), 197-205.

[12] Lu, K. H., & Seidel Jr, G. E. (2004). Effects of heparin and sperm concentration on cleavage and blastocyst development rates of bovine oocytes inseminated with flow cytometrically-sorted sperm. *Theriogenology*, 62(5), 819-30.

[13] Schenk, J. L., Suh, T. K., Cran, D. G., & Seidel Jr, G. E. (1999). Cryopreservation of flow-sorted bovine spermatozoa. *Theriogenology*, 52(8), 1375-91.

[14] Maxwell, W. M. C., Evans, G., Hollinshead, F. K., Bathgate, R., de Graaf, S. P., Eriksson, B. M., et al. (2004). Integration of sperm sexing technology into the ART toolbox. *Animal Reproduction Science*, 82-83, 79-95.

[15] Peippo, J., Vartia, K., Kananen-Anttila, K., Räty, M., Korhonen, K., Hurme, T., et al. (2009). Embryo production from superovulated Holstein-Friesian dairy heifers and

cows after insemination with frozen-thawed sex-sorted X spermatozoa or unsorted semen. *Animal Reproduction Science*, 111(1), 80-92.

[16] Vazquez, J. M., Martinez, E. A., Parrilla, I., Roca, J., Gil, MA, & Vazquez, J. L. (2003). Birth of piglets after deep intrauterine insemination with flow cytometrically sorted boar spermatozoa. *Theriogenology*, 59(7), 1605-14.

[17] Seidel, G. E., & Schenk, J. L. (2008). Pregnancy rates in cattle with cryopreserved sexed sperm: Effects of sperm numbers per inseminate and site of sperm deposition. *Animal Reproduction Science*, 105(1-2), 129-38.

[18] Chebel, R. C., Guagnini, F. S., Santos, J. E. P., Fetrow, J. P., & Lima, J. R. (2010). Sex-sorted semen for dairy heifers: Effects on reproductive and lactational performances. *Journal of dairy science*, 93(6), 2496-507.

[19] Tubman, L. M., Brink, Z., Suh, T. K., & Seidel, G. E. (2004). Characteristics of calves produced with sperm sexed by flow cytometry/cell sorting. *Journal of Animal Science*, 82(4), 1029-36.

[20] Lu, K. H., Cran, D. G., & Seidel Jr, G. E. (1999). In vitro fertilization with flow-cytometrically-sorted bovine sperm. *Theriogenology*, 52(8), 1393-405.

[21] Merton, J. S., de Roos, A. P. W., Mullaart, E., de Ruigh, L., Kaal, L., Vos, P. L. A. M., et al. (2003). Factors affecting oocyte quality and quantity in commercial application of embryo technologies in the cattle breeding industry. *Theriogenology*, 59(2), 651-74.

[22] Xu, J., Guo, Z., Su, L., Nedambale, T. L., Zhang, J., Schenk, J., et al. (2006). Developmental Potential of Vitrified Holstein Cattle Embryos Fertilized In Vitro with Sex-Sorted Sperm. *Journal of dairy science*, 89(7), 2510-8.

[23] De Jarnette, J. M., Mc Cleary, C. R., Leach, M. A., Moreno, J. F., Nebel, R. L., & Marshall, C. E. (2010). Effects of 2.1 and 3.5×106 sex-sorted sperm dosages on conception rates of Holstein cows and heifers. *Journal of Dairy Science*, 93(9), 4079-85.

[24] De Jarnette, J. M., Leach, M. A., Nebel, R. L., Marshall, C. E., Mc Cleary, C. R., & Moreno, J. F. (2011). Effects of sex-sorting and sperm dosage on conception rates of Holstein heifers: Is comparable fertility of sex-sorted and conventional semen plausible? *Journal of Dairy Science*, 94(7), 3477-83.

[25] Borchersen, S., Peacock, M., & Danish, A. I. (2009). field data with sexed semen. *Theriogenology*, 71(1), 59-63.

[26] Seidel Jr, G. E., Schenk, J. L., Herickhoff, L. A., Doyle, S. P., Brink, Z., Green, R. D., et al. (1999). Insemination of heifers with sexed sperm. *Theriogenology*, 52(8), 1407-20.

[27] <Silmerman87-Localization of Luteinizing Hormone-Releasing Hormone (LHRH).pdf>

[28] Sá Filho, M. F., Penteado, L., Reis, E. L., Souza, Reis. T., Galvão, K. N., & Baruselli, P. S. (2012). Timed artificial insemination improves the reproductive performance of suckled beef cows subjected to breeding season. *Theriogenology.;submmited.*

[29] Bodmer, M., Janett, F., Hässig, M., Daas, Nd., Reichert, P., & Thun, R. (2005). Fertility in heifers and cows after low dose insemination with sex-sorted and non-sorted sperm under field conditions. *Theriogenology*, 64(7), 1647-55.

[30] De Jarnette, J. M., Nebel, R. L., & Marshall, C. E. (2009). Evaluating the success of sex-sorted semen in US dairy herds from on farm records. *Theriogenology*, 71(1), 49-58.

[31] Sá Filho, M. F., Girotto, R., Abe, E. K., Penteado, L., Campos, Filho. E. P., Moreno, J. F., et al. (2012). Optimizing the use of sex-sorted sperm in timed artificial insemination programs for suckled beef cows. *Journal of Animal Science*, 90(6), 1816-23.

[32] Mellado, M., Coronel, F., Estrada, A., & Ríos, F. G. (2010). Fertility in Holstein × Gyr cows in a subtropical environment after insemination with Gyr sex-sorted semen. *Tropical Animal Health and Production*, 42(7), 1493-6.

[33] Andersson, M., Taponen, J., Kommeri, M., & Dahlbom, M. (2006). Pregnancy Rates in Lactating Holstein-Friesian Cows after Artificial Insemination with Sexed Sperm. *Reproduction in Domestic Animals*, 41(2), 95-7.

[34] Doyle, S. P., Seidel Jr, G. E., Schenk, J. L., Herickho, L. A., Cran, D. G., & Green, R. D. (1999). Artificial insemination of lactating Angus cows with sexed semen. *American Society of animal Science.*

[35] Hunter, R. H. F. (1994). Causes for failure of fertilization in domestic species. *Zavy MT, Geisert RD, editors. Embryonic Mortality in Domestic Species. Florida: CRC Press, Boca Raton*, 1-22.

[36] Thibault, C. (1973). Sperm transport and storage in vertebrates. *Journal of Reproduction and Fertility*, 18, 39-53.

[37] Hawk, H. W. (1987). Transport and fate of spermatozoa after insemination of cattle. *Journal of dairy science*, 70, 1487-503.

[38] Wilmut, I., & Hunter, R. H. F. (1984). Sperm transport into the oviducts of heifers mated early in oestrus. *Nutrition Development*, 24, 461-8.

[39] Brackett, B. G., Oh, Y. K., Evans, J. F., & Donawick, W. J. (1980). Fertilization and early development of cow ova. 23, 189-205.

[40] Dransfield, M. B. G., Nebel, R. L., Pearson, R. E., & Warnick, L. D. (1998). Timing of Insemination for Dairy Cows Identified in Estrus by a Radiotelemetric Estrus Detection System. *Journal of dairy science*, 81(7), 1874-82.

[41] Roelofs, J. B., van Eerdenburg, F. J. C. M., Soede, N. M., & Kemp, B. (2005). Various behavioral signs of estrous and their relationship with time of ovulation in dairy cattle. *Theriogenology*, 63(5), 1366-77.

[42] Roelofs, J. B., Van Eerdenburg, F. J. C. M., Hazeleger, W., Soede, N. M., & Kemp, B. (2006). Relationship between progesterone concentrations in milk and blood and time of ovulation in dairy cattle. *Animal Reproduction Science*, 91(3-4), 337-343.

[43] Dalton, J. C., & Saacke, R. G. (2007). Parâmetros da qualidade do sêmen para programas de sincronização. *XI Curso Novos Enfoques na Produção e Reprodução de Bovinos; Uberlândia.*

[44] Maatje, K., Loeffler, S. H., & Engel, B. (1997). Optimal time of insemination in cows that show visual signs of estrus by estimating onset of estrus with pedometers. *Journal of dairy science*, 80, 1098-105.

[45] Mee, M. O., Stevenson, J. S., Alexander, B. M., & Sasser, R. G. (1993). Administration of GnRH at estrus influences pregnancy rates, serum concentrations of LH, FSH, estradiol-17 beta, pregnancy-specific protein B, and progesterone, proportion of luteal cell types, and in vitro production of progesterone in dairy cows. *Journal of Animal Science*, 71(1), 185-98.

[46] Kaim, M., Bloch, A., Wolfenson, D., Braw-Tal, R., Rosenberg, M., Voet, H., et al. (2003). Effects of GnRH Administered to Cows at the Onset of Estrus on Timing of Ovulation, Endocrine Responses, and Conception. *Journal of dairy science*, 86(6), 2012-21.

[47] Lee, C. N., Maurice, E., Ax, R. L., Pennington, J. A., Hoffman, W. F., & Brown, M. D. (1983). Efficacy of gonadotropin-releasing hormone administered at the time of artificial insemination of heifers and postpartum and repeat breeder dairy cows. *american journal of veterinary research*, 44, 2160-3.

[48] Perry, G. A., & Perry, B. L. (2009). GnRH treatment at artificial insemination in beef cattle fails to increase plasma progesterone concentrations or pregnancy rates. *Theriogenology*, 71(5), 775-9.

[49] Chenault, J. R., Thatcher, W. W., Kalra, P. S., Abrams, R. M., & Wilcox, C. J. (1975). Transitory Changes in Plasma Progestins, Estradiol, and Luteinizing Hormone Approaching Ovulation in the Bovine. *Journal of dairy science*, 58(5), 709-17.

[50] Rajamahendran, R., & Taylor, C. (1991). Follicular dynamics and temporal relationships among body temperature, oestrus, the surge of luteinizing hormone and ovulation in Holstein heifers treated with norgestomet. *Journal of Reproduction and Fertility*, 92(2), 461-7.

[51] Lucy, M. C., & Stevenson, J. S. (1986). Gonadotropin-releasing hormone at estrus: luteinizing hormone, estradiol, and progesterone during the periestrual and postinsemination periods in dairy cattle. *Biology of Reproduction*, 35(2), 300-11.

[52] Baruselli, P. S., Reis, E. L., Marques, M. O., Nasser, L. F., & Bó, G. A. (2004). The use of hormonal treatments to improve reproductive performance of anestrous beef cattle in tropical climates. *Animal Reproduction Science*, 82, 479-86.

[53] Baruselli, P. S., Ferreira, R. M., Filho, M. F. S., Nasser, L. F. T., Rodrigues, C. A., & Bó, G. A. (2009). Bovine embryo transfer recipient synchronisation and management in tropical environments. *Reproduction, Fertility and Development*, 22(1), 67-74.

[54] Sá Filho, M. F., Torres-Júnior, J. R. S., Penteado, L., Gimenes, L. U., Ferreira, R. M., Ayres, H., et al. (2010). Equine chorionic gonadotropin improves the efficacy of a progestin-based fixed-time artificial insemination protocol in Nelore (Bos indicus) heifers. *Animal Reproduction Science*, 118(2-4), 182-187.

[55] Sá Filho, M. F., Baldrighi, J. M., Sales, J. N. S., Crepaldi, G. A., Carvalho, J. B. P., Bó, G. A., et al. (2011). Induction of ovarian follicular wave emergence and ovulation in progestin-based timed artificial insemination protocols for Bos indicus cattle. *Animal Reproduction Science*, 129(3-4), 132-9.

[56] Carvalho, J. B. P., Carvalho, N. A. T., Reis, E. L., Nichi, M., Souza, A. H., & Baruselli, P. S. (2008). Effect of early luteolysis in progesterone-based timed AI protocols in Bos indicus, Bos indicus×Bos taurus, and Bos taurus heifers. *Theriogenology*, 69(2), 167-75.

[57] Dias, F. C. F., Colazo, M. G., Kastelic, J. P., Mapletoft, R. J., Adams, G. P., & Singh, J. (2010). Progesterone concentration, estradiol pretreatment, and dose of gonadotropin-releasing hormone affect gonadotropin-releasing hormone-mediated luteinizing hormone release in beef heifers. *Domestic Animal Endocrinology*, 39(3), 155-62.

[58] Peres, R. F. G., Júnior, I. C., Filho, O. G. S., Nogueira, G. P., & Vasconcelos, J. L. M. (2009). Strategies to improve fertility in Bos indicus postpubertal heifers and nonlactating cows submitted to fixed-time artificial insemination. *Theriogenology*, 72(5), 681-9.

[59] Baruselli, P. S., Ayres, H., Souza, A. H., Martins, C. M., Gimenes, L. U., & Torres-Júnior, J. R. S. (2006). Impacto da IATF na eficiência reprodutiva em bovinos de corte. *2 Simpósio Internacional de Reprodução Animal Aplicada;; Londrina, PR, Brazil. Faculdade de Medicina Veterinária e Zootecnia da USP*.

[60] Sales, J. N. S., Carvalho, J. B. P., Crepaldi, G. A., Maio, J. R. G., Carvalho, C. A. B., & Barulelli, P. S. (2008). Rate and timing of ovulation in Nelore cows treated with estradiol Cypionate or Benzoate to induce ovulation on FTAI protocols. *reproduction in Domestic Animals*, 43, 181.

[61] Souza, A. H., Sales, J. N. S., Crepaldi, G. A., Teixeira, A. A., & Baruselli, P. S. (2008). Effect of type of semen (sexed vs non-sexed) and time of AI (60h vs 64h) on pregnancy rates of postpartum Nelore cows inseminated in a fixed time. *Animal Reproduction*, 6, 224.

[62] Neves, K. A. L. (2010). Effect of interval between insemination and ovulation in conception rates in Nelore cows timed AI with sex-sorted. *São Paulo: University of São Paulo*.

[63] Sales, J. N. S., Crepaldi, G. A., Fosado, M., Campos, Filho. E. P., & Baruselli, P. S. (2010). Timing of insemination with sexed or nonsexed semen on pregnancy rates of Jersey heifers detected in heat by radiotelemetry. *reproduction fertility and development*, 22, 178.

[64] Seidel, G. E., Allen, C. H., Johnson, L. A., Holland, MD, Brink, Z., Welch, Z. R., et al. (1997). Uterine horn insemination of heifers with very low numbers of nonfrozen and sexed spermatozoa. *Theriogenology*, 48(8), 1255-64.

[65] Underwood, S. L., Bathgate, R., Ebsworth, M., Maxwell, W. M. C., & Evans, G. (2010). Pregnancy loss in heifers after artificial insemination with frozen-thawed, sex-sorted, re-frozen-thawed dairy bull sperm. *Animal Reproduction Science*, 118(1), 7-12.

[66] Soares, J. G., Martins, C. M., Carvalho, N. A. T., Nicacio, A. C., Abreu-Silva, A. L., Campos, Filho. E. P., et al. (2011). Timing of insemination using sex-sorted sperm in embryo production with Bos indicus and Bos taurus superovulated donors. *Animal Reproduction Science*, 127(3-4), 148-53.

[67] Sá Filho, M. F., Santos, J. E. P., Ferreira, R. M., Sales, J. N. S., & Baruselli, P. S. (2011). Importance of estrus on pregnancy per insemination in suckled Bos indicus cows submitted to estradiol/progesterone-based timed insemination protocols. *Theriogenology*, 76(3), 455-63.

[68] Sá Filho, M. F., Crespilho, A. M., Santos, J. E. P., Perry, G. A., & Baruselli, P. S. (2010). Ovarian follicle diameter at timed insemination and estrous response influence likelihood of ovulation and pregnancy after estrous synchronization with progesterone or progestin-based protocols in suckled Bos indicus cows. *Animal Reproduction Science*, 120(1-4), 23-30.

[69] Vazquez, J. M., Parrilla, I., Gil, M. A., Cuello, C., Caballero, I., Vazquez, J. L., et al. (2008). Improving the Efficiency of Insemination with Sex-sorted Spermatozoa. *Reproduction in Domestic Animals*, 43, 1-8.

[70] Olds, D., Seath, D. M., Carpenter, M. C., & Lucas, H. L. (1953). Interrelationships between site of deposition, dosage, and number of spermatozoa in diluted semen and fertility of dairy cows inseminated artificially. *Journal of dairy science*, 36, 1031-5.

[71] Hawk, H. W., & Tanabe, T. Y. (1986). Effect of unilateral cornual insemination upon fertilization rate in superovulating and single-ovulating cattle. *Journal of Animal Science*, 63, 551-60.

[72] Senger, P. L., Becker, W. C., Davidge, S. T., Hillers, J. K., & Reeves, J. J. (1988). Influence of cornual insemination on conception in dairy cattle. *Journal of Animal Science*, 66, 3010-6.

[73] Williams, B. L., Gwazdauskas, F. C., Whittier, W. D., Pearson, R. E., & Nebel, R. L. (1988). Impact of site of inseminate deposition and environmental factors that influence reproduction of dairy cattle. *Journal of dairy science*, 71, 278-83.

[74] Mc Kenna, T., Lenz, R. W., Fenton, S. E., & Ax, R. L. (1990). Nonreturn rates of dairy cattle following uterine body or corneal insemination. *Journal of dairy science*, 73, 1779-83.

[75] Graves, W. M., Dowlen, H. H., Kiess, G. A., & Riley, T. L. (1991). Evaluation of uterine body and bilateral uterine horn insemination techniques. *Journal of dairy science*, 74, 3454-6.

[76] Kurykin, J., Jaakma, Ü., Majas, L., Jalakas, M., Aidnik, M., Waldmann, A., et al. (2003). Fixed time deep intracornual insemination of heifers at synchronized estrus. *Theriogenology*, 60, 1261-8.

[77] Andersson, M., Taponen, J., Koskinen, E., & Dahlbom, M. (2004). Effect of insemination with doses of 2 or 15 million frozen-thawed spermatozoa and semen deposition site on pregnancy rate in dairy cows. *Theriogenology*, 61, 1583-8.

[78] Pallares, A., Zavos, P. M., & Hemken, R. W. (1986). Fertilization rates and embryonic development in superovulated cattle inseminated in different sites within the reproductive tract. *Theriogenology*, 26, 709-19.

Chapter 4

Fertility Results After Artificial Insemination with Bull Semen Frozen with Low Density Lipoprotein Extender

L. Briand-Amirat, D. Bencharif, S. Pineau and D. Tainturier

Additional information is available at the end of the chapter

http://dx.doi.org/10.5772/51868

1. Introduction

The freezing process exposes the spermatozoa to thermal shock, which results in damage to the plasma membrane and acrosome [1, 2]. Various extenders have been tested in an attempt to limit cellular injury. Egg yolk is the most widely used of these extenders by artificial insemination centres. Many demands were formulated to replace egg yolk in extenders by it's cryoprotector factor. In recent years, centrifugation techniques have enabled the isolation of the LDL(Low Density Lipoproteins) that are responsible for the cryopreservative effect of egg yolk [3,4,5]. The incorporation of LDL in bovine extenders has given improved motility results in comparison with extenders containing egg yolk [5,6,7]. However, to extend the use of this new LDL-based extender to insemination centres, a fertility study was essential. Fertility can either be assessed in the laboratory using *in vitro* fertilisation tests or by artificial insemination in the field [8]. The latter provides the most reliable means of assessing semen fertility following freezing and thawing. *In vitro* fertility results have already been published [6]; blastocysts were obtained after 7 days of *in vitro* culture from oocytes collected from abattoirs, matured, and then fertilised *in vitro* with spermatozoa that had been frozen-thawed in the LDL extender. An *in vitro* study is insufficient to assess the fertility of semen that has been frozen in the LDL extender, an *in vivo* field study was therefore necessary.

In vivo fertility of bull semen that had been frozen-thawed in the LDL extender was assessed. A widely available, standard extender (Tris-egg yolk) was used as a control. Cows were thus inseminated with semen that had been frozen-thawed in the LDL extender; pregnancy diagnoses were undertaken to assess the maintenance of fertility.

1.1. Collection of semen, dilution and processing

Two extenders were used; Tris-egg yolk extender (T-EY)): 20 ml of chicken egg yolk and LDL extender: 8% LDL (w/v) in accordance with the method described by Moussa et al. (2002) (patent n° 0100292) [5]. The extenders were thawed on the day of sampling and maintained at 37°C. Three bulls belonging to an artificial insemination centre and that had been approved for public use, were used. All three had a recorded progeny. Using the Laicophos® extender, the artificial insemination centre had a non-return rate at 60-90d of 64.7% for Bull 1, 57.2% for Bull 2, and 72.2% for Bull 3. The semen was collected using an artificial vagina. To excite the bulls, they were teased with a Normandy cow for thirty minutes prior to sampling. The semen was collected into a glass tube that had been previously warmed to 37°C. Following collection, the ejaculates were immediately placed in a water bath at 37°C. Each ejaculate was divided into two equal fractions. Each fraction was immediately diluted to 100 x 10^6 spz/ml with the two extenders that had been previously warmed to 37°C, and then subjected to progressive cooling from 37°C to +4°C over 1h and 30 in a refrigerated unit before being placed into straws. The semen was maintained in equilibrium for 4 hours at +4°C. The straws were held for 10 minutes at +4 cm from the surface of the liquid nitrogen (-120°C) before being immersed and then stored in liquid nitrogen (-196°C).

1.2. Semen evaluation before artificial insemination in the field

Before inseminating the cows, semen was evaluated on motility and plasma membrane integrity. The semen was analysed using the Hamilton-Thorne sperm analyser with the CEROS 12 software program, Hamilton-Thorne biosciences, Inc, Beverly, USA. The machine had been previously configured for the analysis of bovine semen. The following parameters were studied: motility (% mobile spermatozoa), straight line velocity: VSL (µm/sec.), curvilinear velocity: VCL (µm/sec.), the linearity index: LIN (= VSL/VCL x 100), amplitude of lateral head displacement: ALH (µm), and average path velocity: VAP (µm/sec). VAP, VSL, STR, and LIN provide information about the progressive movements of the spermatozoa, VCL and ALH characterise the lateral movements, and BCF (Beat Croix Frequency) provides information about the frequency of movements.

The post-thaw percentage of motile spermatozoa was greater in the LDL extender than in the Tris-egg yolk extender (table 1). The proportion of motile spermatozoa was nearly twice as high in the LDL extender, 58.3% vs. 46% in the Tris-egg yolk (table 1). To evaluate plasma membrane integrity, semen was added to an hypo-osmotic solution (100 mOsm/kg H_2O). The spermatozoa was observed under a phase-contrast microscope and classified as positive or negative. Positive spermatozoa (plasma membrane intact) tail swollen and / or curled:. Negative spermatozoa (plasma membrane damaged) tail not curled. No significant difference (table 2) was found between the semen that had been frozen-thawed in the LDL and Tris-egg yolk extenders. The results of the motility analysis and plasma membrane integrity demonstrated that the semen could be used by stock breeders for artificial insemination.

2. Assesment of in vivo fertility after AI of the cows

One hundred and ninety-three females from 83 different herds were inseminated by three inseminators with 25 years of experience. The females included in the study were from dairy or suckler herds with a Calving to First Insemination Interval (CFI) of more than 60 days, heifers over 18 months old, and first inseminations only. For each insemination, the following data was recorded: date of insemination, herd number, the animal's identification number, breed, lactation or calving index, date of the previous calving if relevant, condition score, the bull used, and the extender used. The pregnancy diagnoses were conducted by recording returns to oestrus and trans-rectal palpation between the 65th and 150th day of gestation. This data is summarised in table 3. Pregnancies can be obtained in the field following the artificial insemination of cows with semen that has been frozen and thawed in the LDL extender. However, no significant difference could be found between the LDL extender and the Tris egg yolk extender in terms of the success rates of insemination (Table 4).

	LDL 8%	Triladyl
Motile spermatozoa (%)	58.3 ± 16.7	46.0 ± 18.2
Rapid (%)	45.3 ± 14.2	27.0 ± 12.3
Average (%)	5.7 ± 3.1	7.7± 2.5
Slow (%)	7.3 ± 3.2	11.3±4.5
Static (%)	43.7 ± 5.5	54.0± 15.1
Hyperactive (%)	5.3 ± 2.1	6.3 ± 5.9
Progressive (%)	34.7 ± 4.0	16.0 ± 6.1
VAP (µm/sec.)	83.5 ± 7.7	71.0 ± 5.3
VSL (µm/sec.)	66.6 ± 9.2	57.3 ± 6.3
LIN (%)	60.7 ± 1.5	58.3± 5.5
STR (%)	82.0 ± 1.7	79.7± 3.2
VCL (µm/sec.)	104.1± 28.6	99.9 ± 5.8
ALH (µm)	4.3 ± 0.3	4.6 ± 1.1

Table 1. Results of the motility of bovine spermatozoa following freezing and thawing in the LDL extender and in the Tris-egg yolk extender obtained using the Hamilton Thorne image analyser (n=3).The results given are the means ± standard deviation of the motility characteristics recorded for the three bulls.

Extender	Total spermatozoa (n)	Swollen spermatozoa (intact) (n) (%)	
LDL 8%	1296	542	41.8
Tris-Egg yolk	1314	559	42.5

Table 2. The effect of LDL and Tris-egg yolk extenders on the integrity of spermatozoal plasma membranes according to the HOS test N = sum of spermatozoa taken from Bulls 1, 2, and 3.

Characteristics of the population		LDL n=98	Tris egg yolk n=95
Breeds	Holstein	n=67	n=81
	Normandy	n=22	n=5
	Charolais	n=7	n=9
	Charolais cross	n=1	
	Aubrac	n=1	
Lactation index	Mean ± standard dev.	1.6 ± 1.9	1.5 ± 1.5
	0	n=29	n=31
	1	n=28	n=24
	2	n=20	n=19
	3	n=9	n=12
	4	n=6	n=5
	"/>4	n=6	n=4
Condition score (mean ± standard deviation)		3.0 ± 0.2	3.0 ± 0.3
Calving to first insemination interval in days (mean ± standard deviation)		94 ± 25 (1 CFI not given)	95 ± 32 (1 CFI not given)

Table 3. Characteristics of the study population for each extender

Extender	Cows inseminated (N)	Positive pregnancy diagnosis	Not pregnant	Success rate at insemination (%)
LDL	98	58	40	59.2
Tris-Egg yolk	95	62	33	65.3

Table 4. Effect of the extender used for freezing the semen on the success rate at insemination (as a %)

3. Is there a correlation between motility and fertility?

Pregnancies were obtained following the artificial insemination of cows with semen that has been frozen-thawed in an LDL extender without any significant difference in the success rate following insemination between the 2 extenders. The initial objective was not to demonstrate the superiority of the LDL extender, but to demonstrate its efficacy in the field in terms of percentage gestation. The success rates with artificial insemination are satisfactory (table 3): 59.2% for the LDL extender and 65.3% for the Tris-egg yolk extender. In a previous study, Amirat et al.2004 [6] demonstrated that fertility was maintained *in vitro*. The hypoosmotic test was chosen to assess plasma membrane integrity as a proven correlation has been found between the results of the HOS test and the *in vivo* fertility rate [9]; the HOS test can therefore be used to predict fertility. Plasma membrane integrity was maintained with both the LDL and Tris-egg yolk extenders (table 2). These results concur with previous studies undertaken in the bovine species [10,11]. Around 60% of the spermatozoa that were frozen-thawed in the LDL extender presented with an alteration of the plasma membrane, whilst around 40% of the spermatozoa lost their motility. The percentage of spermatozoa with an altered plasma membrane may be higher than to the percentage or spermatozoa presenting with a loss of motility. This implies that a certain number of spermatozoa may retain their motility with a damaged plasma membrane, this result agree with that reported by Salamon and Maxwell (1995) [11]. Nevertheless it is unlikely that such spermatozoa would be capable of crossing the zona pellucida.

Motility results demonstrate that the percentage of motile spermatozoa following thawing is superior in the LDL extender in comparison with the Tris-egg yolk extender. These results concur with the works of Moussa et al. (2002) [5] and Amirat et al. (2004) [6]. However, inter-individual variability on the motility performances following thawing has already been reported by Farrell et al. (1998) [12] and Holt (2000) [13]. The results obtained do not make it possible to relate the motility of the spermatozoa to fertility due to the insufficient number of measurements. No study has demonstrated a precise correlation between motility parameters and fertility in cows. In cattle, the percentage of mobile spermatozoa, linearity (LIN), and straight line velocity (VSL) seem to be correlated to fertility according to Budworth et al. (1988) [14], and Farrell et al. (1998)[12]. The average path velocity (VAP), curvilinear velocity (VCL), and the frequency of tail movements (FTM), also appear interesting [12]. According to Liu et al. (1991) [15], the most interesting motility parameters in human semen are linearity (LIN), straight line velocity (VSL), and the percentage of rapid spermatozoa.

4. What parameters could influence the AI success rate?

The confirmation of pregnancies were performed by rectal palpation on average at around the 100th day. However, embryonic mortality is recorded in the same way as failure of fertilisation; this reduces the fertility results observed. Ultrasonographic pregnancy diagnosis at 30 days would have been more accurate for measuring the fertility of the semen as the impact of embryonic mortality is lower between D0 and D30 than between D0 and D150. Descoteaux et al. (2006) [16] thus report that 10% of cows that are given a positive pregnancy diagnosis at 28 days present with embryonic mortality at D60. Nevertheless, the cows included in the present study were selected as a function of various criteria that ensure satisfactory female fertility, which explains the difference in fertility recorded between the results of our study and those reported by Barbat et al. (2005) [17] and Freret et al. (2006) [18]. These studies are based on the results of inseminations conducted over a given period by insemination centres, without any selection criteria for the cows used. Female fertility was therefore inferior to that observed in our study. The observed fertility is a combination of the fertility of the male and female.

In addition to the many different diseases that can affect fertility, other parameters may influence the fertility of cows as breed [17] or lactaction index [19]. In the study described here, the lactation index did not have any significant effect on the overall AI success rate ($p<0.05$). However, the lactation index had an impact for the LDL extender. Superior fertility was observed in the heifers, followed by the primiparous cows. A reduction in fertility was seen in cows with a lactation index of 2 or 3. There were insufficient numbers of cows with high lactation indexes to reveal any trends (Table 6). Milk production [18], energy profile [20], post-partum pathologies [21], and the herd effect [19] are other parameters that interfere with fertility results. Amman and Pickett (1987) [22] show that to measure male fertility a significant number of inseminations are necessary to rule out variations caused by female fertility. Van Wagttendonk de Leeuw et al. (2000) [23] demonstrate that to detect a 2% difference in the non-return rate, with a confidence interval of 95% and a statistical power of 80%, 6,600 inseminations are needed per extender. A limited population of 193 cows was inseminated as it was impossible to undertake a larger scale study due to the difficulty of convincing the breeders to use semen that had been frozen and thawed in an extender that did not have proven *in vivo* efficacy. The population was divided into two relatively homogeneous groups (mean lactation index, condition score, CFI) to limit variations in female fertility. The inclusion criteria could be improved: it would have been judicious to use only one breed to limit interbreed fertility differences [17]. It would also have been preferable for all of the cows to have the same lactation index. The milk production of the animals affects their fertility [18]. The latter was not recorded as some of the farmers in this study did not keep individual milk production records. The use of condition scoring enables any animals that are in negative energy balance to be excluded [24]. The bulls were chosen on the basis of good individual fertility and on the presence of the bulls at the centre at the time of semen collection. The bull factor did not exert any significant difference ($p<0.05$) on the total insemination success rate (Table 5). The bull effect was observed in the sub-population of cows that had been inseminated with the semen that had been frozen-thawed in the LDL extender ($p=0.019$). The semen from bull 2 that had been frozen in Tris-egg yolk was significantly more fertile than that which had been frozen in the LDL ($p=0.046$). The variation in success for bull 3 was due to the small number of cows inseminated. The cows were taken from numerous farms and we did not al-

http://dx.doi.org/10.5772/51868

ways have intra-herd paired animals: the herd effect could not therefore be assessed. In this study, fewer constraints were voluntary imposed on the inclusion criteria as many animals as possible in order to facilitate the task of the inseminators.

The inseminator did not have a significant influence on the total Insemination Success Rate, with a threshold of significance of p=0.05 (Table 5). Inseminator 3 achieved higher insemination success rates for both extenders McKenna et al. (1990) [25] calculated the inseminator effect at ± 9.5 points. The animals that he inseminated were on average younger with a higher proportion of heifers. Barbat et al. (2005) [17] reported superior fertility in heifers in comparison with cows.

Percentage success at insemination (%)	**Inseminator 1**		**Inseminator 2**		**Inseminator 3**		**TOTAL**
extender	LDL	T.E.Y	LDL	T.E.Y	LDL	T.E.Y	
Bull 1	25.0(*),(**)	83.3(*)	72.2(**)	60.0	87.5(**)	62.5	82
	n=12	n=12	n=11	n=15	n=16	n=16	
Bull 2	38.5	73.3	36.4	41.7	50.0	90.0	71
	n=13	n=15	n=11	n=12	n=10	n=10	
Bull 3	88.2	50.0	50.0	25.0	50.0	100.0	40
	n=17	n=8	n=2	n=4	n=6	n=3	
TOTAL	54.8	71.4	54.2	48.4	68.7	75.8	**193**
	n=42	n=35	n=24	n=31	n=32	n=31	

*: significant difference between the two extenders for Bull 1 when the insemination was performed by inseminator 1 (p=0.002)

**: significant difference between the inseminators for Bull 1 with the LDL extender (p= 0.004)

Table 5. Insemination success rate (in %), details of the bulls and inseminators for each of the extenders, LDL and Tris Egg Yolk (TEY)

Lactation index	LDL	Tris egg yolk	Total AI success rates
0	82.8(*)	61.3	71.6
	n=29	n=31	n=60
1	53.6(*)	75.0	63.5
	n=28	n=24	n=52
2 and 3	37.9(*)	61.3	50.0
	n=29	n=31	n=60
≥4	66.7(*)	66.7	66.7
	n=12	n=9	n=21

*: significant difference in the lactation index for the 8% LDL extender (p=0.005)

Table 6. Insemination success rates (in %) as a function of the lactation index

5. Conclusion

Although semen fertility was difficult to measure due to the various parameters that intervene causing variations in the results, this preliminary study enabled us to demonstrate for the first time that bull semen that has been frozen then thawed in the LDL extender retains a good level of fertility since gestations were obtained following artificial insemination. The continuation of this study in a larger population would make it possible to specify the impact of the LDL extender on the success of artificial insemination.

Author details

L. Briand-Amirat*, D. Bencharif, S. Pineau and D. Tainturier

Laboratory of Biotechnology and Pathology of Reproduction, Nantes Atlantic College of Veterinary Medicine,
Food Science and Engineering, Nantes, France

References

[1] Woelders H, Matthijs A, Engel B. Effects of trehalose and sucrose, osmolality of the freezing medium, and cooling rate on viability and intactness of bull sperm after freezing and thawing, Cryobiology 1997;35:93-105.

[2] Celeghini, E.C.C.; Arruda, R.P.; Andrade, A.F.C.; Nascimento, J.; Raphael, C.F.; Rodrigues, P.H.M. Effects that bovine sperm cryopreservation using two different extenders has on sperm membranes and chromatin. Animal Reproduction Science 2007; 100: 1-13.

[3] Pace M M, Graham E F. Components in egg yolk which protect bovine spermatozoa during freezing. J Anim Sci 1974; 39: 1144-1149.

[4] Demianowicz W, Strezek J. The effect of lipoprotein fraction of egg yolk on some of the biological properties of boar spermatozoa during storage of the semen in liquid state. Reprod Dom Anim 1996; 31: 279-280

[5] Moussa M, Martinet V, Trimeche A, Tainturier D, Anton M. Low density lipoproteins extracted from hen egg yolk by an easy method: cryoprotective effect on frozen-thawed bull semen. Theriogenology 2002;57:1695-1706

[6] Amirat L, Tainturier D, Jeanneau L, Thorin C, Gérard O, Courtens JL, Anton M. Bull semen in vitro fertility after cryopreservation using egg yolk LDL: a comparison with Optidyl, a commercial egg yolk extender. Theriogenology 2004; 61:895-907.

[7] Vera Munoz O, Amirat-Briand L, Diaz T, Vasquez L, Schmidt E, Desherces S, Anton M, Bencharif D, Tainturier D. Effect of semen dilution to low-sperm number per dose on motility and functionality of cryopreserved bovine spermatozoa using low-density lipoproteins (LDL) extender : Comparison to Triladyl and Bioxcell. Theriogenology 2009, 71: 895-900

[8] Larsson B, Rodriguez-Martinez H. Can we use in vitro fertilization tests to predict fertility ? Anim reprod Sci 2000; 60/61:327-336.

[9] Brito LF, Barth AD, Bilodeau-Goeseeis S, Panich PL, Kastelic JP. Comparison of methods to evaluate the plasmalemma of bovine sperm and their relationship with *in vitro* fertilization rate. Theriogenology 2003;60:1539-51

[10] Correa JR, Rodriguez MC, Patterson DJ, Zavos PM. Thawing and processing of cryopreserved bovine spermatozoa at various temperatures and their effects on sperm viability, osmotic shock and sperm membrane functional integrity. *Theriogenology,* 1996; 46(3), 413-420

[11] Salamon S, Maxwell WMC. Frozen storage of ram semen. II. Causes of low fertility after cervical insemination and methods of improvement. Anim Reprod Sci 1995;381-36.

[12] Farrel PB, Presicce GA, Brockett CC, Foote RH. Quantification of bull sperm characteristics measured by computer-assisted sperm analysis (C.A.S.A.) and the relationship to fertility. *Theriogenology,* 1998, 49, 871-879

[13] Holt WV. Fundamental aspects of sperm cryobiology: the importance of the species and individual differences. *Theriogenology,* 2000; 53(1), 47-58

[14] Budworth PR, Amann RP, Chapman PL. Relationship between computerized measurements of motion of frozen-thawed bull spermatozoa and fertility. *Journal of Andrology* 1988, 9, 41-54.

[15] Liu DY, Clarke GN, Gordon Baker HW. Relationship between sperm motility assessed with the Hamilton-Thorn Motility Analyser and fertilisation rates in vitro. *Andrology.* 1991, 12, 231-239

[16] Descôteaux L, Carrière PD, Durochet J. Ultrasonography of the reproductive system of the cow : basic principles, practical uses and economic aspects of the diagnostic tool in dairy production. 24th World Buiatrics Congress, Nice, 2006, p303-310

[17] Barbat A, Druet T, Bonati B, Guillaume F, Colleau JJ, Boichard D. Bilan phénotypique de la fertilité à l'insémination artificielle dans les trois principales races françaises. Renc. Rech. Ruminants. 2005, 137-140

[18] Freret S, Ponsart C, Rai DB, Jeanguyot N, Paccard P, Humblot P. Facteurs de variation de la fertilité en première insémination et des taux de mortalités embryonnaires en élevages laitiers Prim'Holstein. Renc. Rech. Rum. 2006, 281-284

[19] Seegers H, Beaudeau F, Blosse A, Ponsart C, Humblot P. Performances de reproduction aux inséminations de rangs 1 et 2 dans les troupeaux Prim'holstein. Renc. Rech. Rum. 2005, 141-144

[20] Domecq JJ, Skidmore A L, Lloyd J W, Kaneene J B. Relationship between body condition scores and conception at first artificial insemination in a large dairy herd of high yielding Holstein cows. *J. Dairy Sci.* 1997, 80(1), 113-120

[21] Hanzen C, Pluvinage P. Stress et performances de reproduction. *Le Point Vétérinaire.* 2005, 36, 94-98

[22] Amman RP, Pickett BW. Principles of cryopreservation and a review of cryopreservation of stallion spermatozoa. Equine Vet. Sci. 1987, 7, 145-173

[23] Van Wagtendonk-de Leeuw A M, Haring R M, Kaal-Lansbergen L M T E, Den Daas J H G : Fertility results using bovine semen cryopreserved with extenders based on egg yolk and soy bean extract. *Theriogenology.* 2000, 54(1), 57-67

[24] Grimard B, Humblot P, Ponter A A, Mialot J P, Sauvant D, Thibier M. Influence of postpartum energy restriction on energy status, plasma LH and oestradiol secretion and follicular development in suckled beef cows. *J Reprod Fertil.* 1995, 104(1), 173-179

[25] McKenna T, Lenz R W, Fenton SE., Ax RL. : Nonreturn Rates of Dairy Cattle Following Uterine Body or Cornual Insemination. *J. Dairy Sci.* 1990, 73(7), 1779-1783

Chapter 5

Nonsteroid Anti-Inflammatory Drugs to Improve Fertility in Cows

Zahid Paksoy and Hüseyin Daş

Additional information is available at the end of the chapter

http://dx.doi.org/10.5772/51910

1. Introduction

The bulk of milk production in the world is supplied from the cows. Besides the fact that genetic is the most important factor in a cow's milk productivity; feeding and environmental factors are also considered as crucial factors. Because of these points, calving and increasing reproductive performance has become the most fundamental issue for milk industry. For the animal breeders both having milk and obtaining a calf throughout a year is indispensable. To accomplish this, there should not be a problem in a herd from the aspect of reproduction. But many factors like diseases and environmental agents in cows in post partum period cause decrease in fertility. Among the reasons of reduction in fertility; there are factors like indetermination of estrus in time or detection of estrus in wrong time, premature estrus, subestrus, anestrus, delaying of ovulation, failure of ovulation and fertilization, inadequacy of communication between embryo and uterus, poor body condition score, heat stress, dystocia, retained placenta, delayed uterine involution, metritis, endometritis, and other illnesses. Although a great deal of studies has been done to lower the infertility caused by these factors, this problem has not been eradicated completely up to these days [1-6].

The reasons mentioned above are associated with female animals and environmental conditions. Together with this, fertility is dependent not only to the female but also to the male. There should not be a problem in male's genital organs and the male must have the ability to produce sperms to fertilize the ovum. If artificial insemination is carried out, morphologic structures, numbers, motilities of the sperms should be normal [7-10].

Progestagens and Prostaglandin F_2 alpha ($PGF_2\alpha$) have been used to prevent the disorders related to estrus. But observation of estrus is necessary in both administrations. For this reason researchers have dealt with developing protocols without estrus observation. Ovulations have been synchronized with a method developed in Wisconsin University, and this method was named as Ovsynch. Later, this method has been modified by the combined use of both progestagens and prostaglandins and many modified ovsynch protocols have been derived [11-12].

Nowadays, one of the methods used by the veterinarians to increase the percentage of pregnancy in cows is GnRH and hCG application just before the artificial insemination, together with the insemination or 1st – 15th days after insemination because hormonal balance is very crucial in early embryonic period. Nearly, 25% of cattle embryos die within the first three weeks of pregnancy [4, 13-15]. In this period, continuation of progesterone release by corpus luteum is vital for the life of embryo [16]. For this reason, researchers have strived to keep the progesterone level sufficient enough in early pregnancy by administering GnRH and hCG in different days of estrus cycle. hCG application is done to animals during the insemination or luteal period in order to provide the rupture of Graafian follicle, to abolish functional insufficiencies of corpus luteum and to rise the endogenous progesterone production to the most effective level, and as a result of these applications it has been stated that pregnancy rate has increased in some studies [17-18]. In the same way, with the GnRH application before, during and post insemination in different days, it has been notified that pregnancy rate has been increased by means of stimulating folliculogenesis, ovulation and luteal structures [19-21].

The latest method to regulate maternal and fetal relation, to retard or inhibit luteolysis, to maintain high progesterone levels and as a result; to enhance pregnancy rate is application of Nonsteroid Anti-inflammatory Drugs (NSAID) in critical days of pregnancy. Estrus cycle's hormonal mechanism should be very well known for the good management of this process.

2. Estrus cycle

Cows are polyestrous animals throughout the year. They show estrus within 18-24 day periods only if they are not pregnant. Estrus cycle is controlled and managed by hormones released by hypothalamus, hypophysis, ovaries and uterus [22].

In the start of estrus cycle GnRH plays the most important role [23]. By giving GnRH released from hypothalamus in each 30 – 120 minute periods to hypophysis system, it induces synthesis and release of Follicle Stimulating Hormone (FSH) and Luteinizing Hormone (LH). With the FSH effect follicles in the ovaries start to grow. Follicular development is observed in waves. In each wave just one follicle passes to dominant state from the many developed follicles, rarely two follicles passes to preovulatory stage. Follicular development or atresia is not seen in other follicles in follicular wave. While estradiol produced from preovulatory follicle induces LH release, it inhibits FSH release [3, 5, 24]. But FSH release is not only regulated by estradiol and GnRH, inhibin which is an ovary originated peptide also inhibits FSH release just like estradiol. Moreover, activin which is a peptide hormone found in follicular liquid induces FSH release, but follistatin inhibits it [5].

Released estrogen both causes physiological changes in genital canal and emergence of overt estrus signs. Ovulation in cows takes place 24 to 30 hours after the peak of LH. Ovulated follicle undergoes structural and functional change with the effect of LH and metamorphoses to corpus luteum. Developing corpus luteum releases progesterone, and so, it makes a negative feedback to hypothalamus and by hindering FSH and LH release it also follicular activities in ovaries. In the meantime, by inhibiting contractions of uterus and stimulating the glands in endometrium, it causes the liquid so called uterus milk to be released. As a result it prepares a suitable ambient and provides the continuation of gestation [5, 22, 25-28].

If there is not a live embryo in uterus in the 16th -18th days of cycle, $PGF_2\alpha$ is synthesized, and causes the corpus luteum's regression and decreases the progesterone secretion. Decrease in progesterone causes LH peak and this increase in LH results in increase of estradiol level. While luteolysis is progressing, a new preovulatory follicle develops and cycle resumes. If the animal gets pregnant, $PGF_2\alpha$ secretion is blocked and progesterone level stays in the level enough for sustain the gestation [16, 24, 25, 27].

3. Fertilisation

Gestation is a process which starts with fertilisation and completed with birth of the young. Fertilization is the name given to the event of forming a diploid chromosome cell from two haploid chromosome cells by entering of spermatozoon into oocyte [29].

Fertilization takes place in oviduct ampulla in domestic mammals. It happens approximately in 12 hours. In the end, zygote forms [30-31].

4. Early embryonic period

Zygote undergoes a set of mitotic division which is called "segmentation". With the first segmentation division, blastomere which is a two cell embryo forms. When the blastomeres proliferate in countless numbers it is called morula. Then, water diffusion starts in morula and a liquid filled blank which is called blastocele forms. When this blank forms, embryo is called as blastocyte [30, 32].

When blastocyte undergoes a mitotic division, liquid continues to accumulate in the blastocele and for this reason pressure inside the embryo increases. Proteolytic enzymes and blastocyte contraction and relaxation movements cause the tear of zona pelucida. When there is a little tear in zona pellucida, blastocyte goes out. This prolapsus which is called as hatching takes place between 9th and 11th days in cows. After this stage, embryo lives freely in uterus until implantation and feeds with uterus milk [14, 24, 30, 32].

15th to 17th days of the gestation is considered as the critical period. Embryonic deaths taking place in this stage causes dramatic economic losses. During this period, unless the signal to prevent the production of $PGF_2\alpha$ is sent, endometrial luteolytic $PGF_2\alpha$ release will be realized. For the continuation of gestation this endometrial $PGF_2\alpha$ production must be hindered. Biology of this critical period is complex and affected from very different events. Forming of luteolysis or continuation of gestation is dependent on hormonal, cellular and molecular factors belonging to both mother and the embryo. In order to increase the pregnancy rate in artificial insemination and embryo transfer, hCG, eCG and GnRH applications are done in this critical period. In these applications, while increasing progesterone amount, decreasing plasma estradiol 17 beta amounts and inhibiting $PGF_2\alpha$ synthesis from endometrium is aimed [16].

5. Embryo signals and pregnancy recognition

Blockage of luteolysis during the recognition of gestation can be possible by inhibition of estradiol production because existence of estradiol is obligatory for luteolysis. Estradiol induces $PGF_2\alpha$ secretion. When compared with cyclic animals, follicular development and concentration of plasma estradiol are less in pregnant animals. How does estradiol affects $PGF_2\alpha$ secretion in cellular and molecular levels is not known. However, estradiol has got a central role in luteolysis. For this reason; while antilteolytic strategies are developed, for the retardation or inhibition of luteolysis decrease of estradiol level is aimed [16].

Progesterone amount circulating in cows provides maternal recognition. This situation shows the importance of high level progesterone for the recognition of pregnancy in critical period. Another factor for the pregnancy recognition is bovine interferon-tau which is released by the embryo. Bovine interferon-tau is also known as bovine trophoblast protein-1 (bTP-1). Bovine interferon-tau which is secreted to lumen of uterus inhibits the release of $PGF_2\alpha$ from the endometrium in critical period. Stimulating of progesterone to bovine interferon-tau is another possible mechanism for the maternal recognition. In the cows, which have higher levels of progesterone in the critical period, more bovine interferon-tau is produced by the embryo [16, 32].

Interferon-tau shows its affect by hindering estradiol receptors. Subsequently, oxytocin receptors diminish and cyclooxygenase inhibitors get activated. Interferon-tau insures the production of some endometrial proteins crucial for the life of embryo. The first of these proteins is bovine granulocyte protein-2. Second one is ubiquitin cross-reactive protein (UCRP). UCRP conjugates with cytosolic endometrial proteins in response to pregnancy and interferon-tau. Proteins conjugated with UCRP become a target for processing by proteasome. This affect of interferon-tau is mediated by the induction of signal transducer and activation of transcription 1 (STAT-1), STAT-2, and interferon regulatory factor 1. UCRP, alpha chemokines and induction of these transcription factors procure pregnancy recognition by mother [33].

6. Early embryonic death

Embryonic death is the most important source of reproductive losses. During the first three weeks of pregnancy embryonic deaths occur by means of several factors. If embryonic deaths take place between the 24th and 50th days, it is called as late embryonic death [4, 13].

Even in healthy cows in the first three weeks of pregnancy, more than 25% of the embryos cannot continue its development. While fertilization rate in cows with first service is 90%, calving rate is about 50-60% [4, 14]. In a study associated with this topic, it is reported that calving rate is 70% after insemination and most of the 30% of embryo losses take place in between 6th and 18th days [34]. If embryonic death happens before 16th - 17th days, cows continue to show estrus within normal intervals. However, if embryonic death happens after 16th - 17th days, returning back to estrus cycle takes longer and cycle interval becomes irregular [4].

There are plenty of factors that cause embryonic death in cows. These are; endocrine, genetic, intrinsic and extrinsic environmental factors, climate, stress, age, insemination time, semen quality, infectious agents, nutrition, chromosomal anomalies. Especially, abnormal progesterone and estrogen profiles cause embryonic deaths. Moreover, in high producing cows steroid metabolism is faster because of liver blood circulation increase. And this causes lower levels of progesterone in luteal period of estrus cycle [4, 35].

7. Embryonic losses due to endocrinologic causes

Low progesterone levels lead to death of embryo by causing excessive estradiol and $PGF_2\alpha$ secretion. It is required that luteolytic effects of estradiol and $PGF_2\alpha$ should be decreased in the early period after insemination in order for maternal recognition of pregnancy [36].

Researchers assert that low progesterone concentration before insemination period causes abnormal follicular development, elicit abnormal oocyte development in ovulatory follicle and ultimately, it causes early embryonic death [37-38].

Adequate secretion of progesterone in luteal period is vital for healthy ovulation, nutrition and survival of developing embryo. Low level of progesterone leads to embryonic death for reasons of:

1. Low progesterone levels from ovulation to 6th day after the insemination causes the inhibition of embryo's development.
2. If progesterone is insufficient in pre-estrus period, uterus deprives of progesterone receptors. As a result of this, in 4th – 9th days of post insemination excessive $PGF_2\alpha$ secretion forms, and this makes both an embryotoxic and luteolytic affect.
3. In 14th – 17th days which are the days of pregnancy recognition, cause of low pregnancy rate is progesterone inadequacy and excessiveness of estradiol.
4. Low progesterone levels in late embryonic period indicate imminent embryonic death [36, 39].

Oxytocin produced by corpus luteum stimulates the release of $PGF_2\alpha$ from endometrium. $PGF_2\alpha$ production depends on reaching of oxytocin receptor number to a threshold value. When these receptors in endometrium reaches a sufficient number, pulsatil secretion of

$PGF_2\alpha$ occurs in response to luteal oxytocin secretion and luteolysis goes after. For this reason, maternal recognition of pregnancy must take place before luteolysis [32, 40].

Specific proteins (bTP-1) produced by blastocyst in cows are signals preventing luteolysis. bTP-1, inhibits the endometrium cells' oxytocin receptor production. As a result, oxytocin cannot induce $PGF_2\alpha$ release. In addition to this, bTP-1increases protein production from uterine glands. These released proteins into uterus lumen provide nutrition of embryo [32].

8. Cyclooxygenase – COX (Prostaglandin endoperoxide synthase)

NSAIDs[1] are the most commonly used drugs for the treatment of pain for centuries. These drugs also have antipyretic and analgesic affects. They act by inhibiting the enzyme cyclooxygenase (also known as Cox inhibitors). In this way, the synthesis of prostaglandins is blocked. Prostaglandins are mediators which ensure the formation of inflammation symptoms as pain, fever and swelling. Arachidonic acid, which is found in cell membrane, is precursor of prostaglandins. Prostaglandins are end products of fatty acid metabolism. With the effect of Phospholipase A_2, Arachidonic acid is synthesized from membrane phospholipids. As soon as arachidonic acid is released Prostaglandin G_2 and Prostaglandin H_2 is synthesized by the effect of cox enzyme. Then, by means of synthase, PGD_2, PGE_2, PGF_2, PGI_2 and TxA_2 are produced [41-45]. See figure 1.

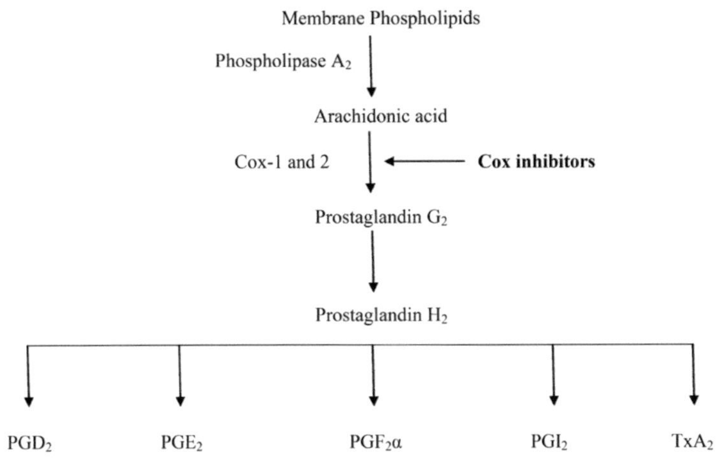

Figure 1. Metabolism of Prostaglandins.

Nowadays, the most known NSAID is aspirin. The past of Aspirin dates back to hundreds of years. The most important step in the discovery of Aspirin is the identification of salicylic acid in 1860. Following this discovery, sodium salicylate in 1875 and phenyl salicylate in

1 NSAID: Nonsteroid Anti-inflammatory Drugs

1886 were first used. But these drugs formed serious side effects in gastrointestinal system. Aspirin or acetyl salicylic acid was discovered by Felix Hoffman in 1897. It was started to be sold under the name of Aspirin by Bayer Company in 1899 [46].

For the first time, it has been identified that prostaglandin inhibitors prevent product of Cox by John Vane in 1971 [44]. Later studies have shown that Cox enzymes have different isoforms and have different functions. Cox-1 is found in stomach, intestine, kidney and thrombocytes, and Cox-2 is secreted in platelets, macrophages, endothelial cells [41, 47]. While classic NSAIDs inhibit both enzymes, Cox-2 inhibitors inhibit inducible Cox-2. Thanks to this, Cox-2 inhibitors can show anti-inflammatory effect without forming any side effects in gastrointestinal system and in other tissues [43]. Existence of Cox-3 enzyme was discovered by Chandrasekharan et al. in 2002 [48]. See table 1.

Class	Active Ingredient	Effect
Cox-1 Specific Agents	Low Dose Aspirin	It makes COX-1 inhibition without doing COX-2 inhibition.
COX Non-specific Agents	Diclofenac, Ketorolak, Asetaminofen, Flunixin meglumine.	It inhibits both enzymes.
COX-2 Selective Agents	Meloxicam, Nabumetane, Nimesulid, Carpofren.	With Clinic threpautic doses in human and animals, while doing COX-2 inhibition, in increasing doses they cause COX-1 inhibition.
COX-2 Specific Agents	Celecoxib, Rofecoxib.	They are agents which do not cuase COX-1 inhibition even in maximum threpautic clinical doses.

Table 1. Cox inhibitors are classified as below [41, 49]:

Cox inhibitors are used with different aims in reproductive field. Among these are; blocking of ovulation and implantation, preventing post operative adhesions and hindering of premature births (tocolytic) [50-58].

A lot of studies have been done to understand the importance of Cox enzyme in implantation. It has been found out that COX-2 is produced by uterus luminal epithel and stroma which surround blastocyte during implantation in rats. This situation indicates that COX-2 has a fundamental role in implantation [59-60]. Again in another study, it has been identified that female rats which have COX-1 deficiency have normal fertility and young number. Because in the presence of COX-1 enzyme deficiency, COX-2 supplies this deficit [59]. However, female rats which have COX-2 deficiency are infertile. Because lacking of COX-2 enzyme occurs ovulation, fertilization, implantation and desidualization defects [61].

Parallel with the studies done on experiment animals, studies searching the effects of NSAIDs on pregnancy rates of livestock have also been done. In these studies, flunixin meglumine, meloxicam, and carprofen have been used in order to increase pregnancy rate in cows.

9. Flunixin meglumine

Flunixin meglumine is a derivation of nicotinic acid and is also a non-selective cox inhibitor. It is a potent NSAID to keep the inflammation, pain and fever under control. Especially, it is used in visceral pains. In addition to its analgesic effect, it has antiendotoxic and antipyretic effects. Flunixin meglumine's half-life is between 8 and 12 hours in cows, but it is longer in other animals [49, 62].

Flunixin meglumine is used in cows combined with antibiotics to cure illnesses like; joint ill, transit fever, blackleg, superfoul, mastitis, puerperal metritis, vaginal prolapse, pneumonia, downer cow. Moreover, it is used in pain therapy after small operations [63-64].

Flunixin meglumine is used in cows in ways like intramuscular, intravenous and peros. When it is used orally, the dose is 1 mg/kg. 1.1-2.2 mg/kg dose is used in intravenous way. The most application way is intramuscular injection and the dose is 1.1 mg/kg. This dose of flunixin meglumine is given once in a day or two times by dividing the dose. Flunixin meglumine can be given in 6-8 hour intervals in 0.25-0.50 mg/kg doses. Average therapy period is three days and it can be given 5 days maximum [65-69].

10. Carprofen

Carprofen is a propionic acid derivative NSAID and a selective cox-2 inhibitor. The drugs in this group take –fen suffix (e.g. ibuprofen, ketoprofen). Carprofen is the safest drug in this group because its peripheral prostaglandin inhibition is weak. It is a long effective NSAID with a clinical effect time of 12 hours. Carprofen in cows administered subcutaneous, in dose of 1.4 mg/kg to body weight [49, 65, 70-72].

11. Meloxicam

Meloxicam is a selective cox-2 inhibitor. It is an oxicam group NSAID. It has anti-inflammatory, analgesic and antipyretic effects. Half-life is 13 hours in cows. It is used in cows by intramuscular, intravenous and subcutaneous ways in single doses of 0.5 mg/kg [65, 70-71].

12. NSAID use after insemination

In many studies about usage of flunixin meglumine, carprofen and meloxicam in different times after post insemination, decreasing $PGF_2\alpha$ release, increasing luteal progesterone level and preventing early embryonic deaths are aimed [72-75].

In some of these studies [74-77], deserved pregnancy rates have been accomplished, on the other hand in some other studies [78-80] pregnancy rates have not changed.

In a study [75], in order to prevent early embryonic deaths in cows which are exposed to transportation stress, flunixin meglumine was given. In the study animals were divided into 3 groups as; control, stress (S) and stress +flunixin meglumine (SFM). After the synchronization of the cows' estrus with MGA - $PGF_2\alpha$, insemination was done by observing the estrus. Animals were exposed to stress 14 days after the insemination. 1.1 mg/kg dose of flunixin meglumine was given to SFM group before transportation. Just transportation stress was formed in S group. When looked at the pregnancy rates (Control 76%, Stress 69% and SFM 84%), it is seen that there is a positive relation between pregnancy rates and flunixin meglumine application.

Merrill et al [76] searched the effects of 1.1mg/kg dose of flunixin meglumine administration on embryonic mortality of stressful and unstressed cows. They used 259 heifers and 127 cows. They designed the application groups as; control, control + flunixin meglumine, stress and stress + flunixin meglumine. In the first experiment, they used 259 angus crossbred heifers. All the heifers were synchronized with Controlled Internal Drug-Release (CIDR®) and $PGF_2\alpha$. In the second experiment, they used 127 angus crossbred cows. All the cows were synchronized with MGA and $PGF_2\alpha$. Applications started 14 days after artificial insemination. While pregnancy rate of animals exposed to transportation stress is 62%, unstressed animals had 64% pregnancy rate. While the pregnancy rate of flunixin meglumine cured animals was 69%, it was 59% in others. In the first experiment they reported that flunixin meglumine given animals had more pregnancy rate than others which were not given. In the second experiment, it was reported that flunixin meglumine applied animals had higher pregnancy rates than others (80% vs. 66%).

In another study, single dose of flunixin meglumine injection (1.1 mg/kg) was done on the 14th day after the insemination to animals which were exposed to transportation stress. The effect of this application on early embryonic deaths and prostaglandin in circulation and cortisol levels were searched. Researchers used 483 beef cows and animals were divided into 4 groups. They designed the groups as; first group transport, second group transport + flunixin meglumine, third group no transport (n=130) and the last group no transport + flunixin meglumine. After the application, transport + flunixin meglumine group had higher pregnancy rate than flunixin meglumine free group (74% vs. 66%) without looking at transportation. Just flunixin meglumine administered cows' pregnancy rates were found higher than non-flunixin meglumine cows (71% vs. 61%). Cortisol concentration in cows exposed to transportation stress got increased but pregnancy rate did not change. In flunixin meglumine given subjects prostaglandin concentration was found lower than not givens. As a result researchers came to conclusion that NSAID applications would increase the pregnancy rate [77] .

Odensvik et al [81] have reported that application of flunixin meglumine both orally and parentally supports luteal function. They administered 2, 3 or 4 oral doses 2.2 mg/kg flunixin meglumine to heifers. They started the 9 day-therapy period 14-15 days of the estrus. As a result, they have found that estrus cycle is prolonged in groups of 3 and 4 doses administration. Luteolysis have taken place when 2 or 3 doses of flunixin meglumine have been applied. But in 4 dose give groups luteolysis have been postponed. The first cycle of the animals was evaluated as control and the 2nd cycle was evaluated as therapy cycle. Before the experiment, cycles of the animals were synchronized by $PGF_2\alpha$.

Dogruer et al. [82] synchronized repeat breeder heifers by applying two dose $PGF_2\alpha$. 48 hours after $PGF_2\alpha$, they administered GnRH (buserelin acetate) and after 12 – 14 hours they made fixed time artificial insemination. Then, they divided the heifers into two groups randomly and they injected a group flunixin meglumine on the 15th and 16th days. They used the other group as control. They made a pregnancy test to animals on the 29th day and in the end, they identified 50% pregnancy rate in therapy group, and 20% in the control group.

Güzeloğlu et al [74] gave GnRH on the 48th hour after synchronisation with $PGF_2\alpha$ to 52 Holstein heifers and they inseminated them after 12-14 hours. Following this application, they administered 1.1 mg/kg dose of flunixin meglumine after artificial insemination on 15th days evening and 16th days morning via intramuscular way. Pregnancy test was done on the 29th day and, 20 pregnant animals in the treatment group and 13 pregnant animals in the control group was found.

In a study by Lucacin et al [78], they administered 1.1 mg/kg dose of flunixin meglumine to animals between the estrus cycle's 11th and 16th days. Saline solution was given to animals in the control group. The estrus cycle of the animals was synchronized by the applications of estradiol benzoate + CIDR + $PGF_2\alpha$ and then, fixed time artificial insemination was done. Researchers did not find any difference between progesterone concentrations and pregnancy rates of treatment group and control group.

Rabaglino et al. [79] synchronized the heifers with Cosynch+CIDR protocol, they gave half of them double dose of flunixin meglumine (400 mg) on the 15th and 16th days after artificial insemination. At the end of this application, 59.4% pregnancy was reached in control group, 59.5% pregnancy rate was reached in Flunixin meglumine given group.

Geary et al. [80] searched the effects of flunixin meglumine on the pregnancy rates in a study done on Angus heifers. In the first experiment they synchronized the animals with MGA and $PGF_2\alpha$. Animals were inseminated 12 hours after the observation of estrus. 13 days after the artificial insemination they injected single dose of flunixin meglumine to animals. While pregnancy rate was 72% in control group, it remained 66% in flunixin meglumine group. In the second experiment, Angus cows were synchronized via Select Synch or Select Synch + CIDR method. After that, they were inseminated by observing estrus. Around 13 days after artificial insemination they were injected flunixin meglumine. In the pregnancy test done on the 47th day, no difference was observed between the control and subject group (57% vs. 58%). In the third experiment both the heifers and the cows were used as materials. While Heifers were synchronized through Select Synch + CIDR protocol, cows were synchronized with Co-Synch + CIDR protocol. Pregnancy test was done on the 29th day; it was confirmed on the 75th day in heifers and 99th day in cows by ultrasound examination. As the conclusion of the experiment, no difference was found between flunixin meglumine and control group (50% vs. 48%).

Kruger and Heuwiser [83] made a study to assess the carprofen and flunixin meglumine's effect on pregnancy rate of dairy cattle. They injected animals with carprofen and flunixin meglumine on 14th, 15th and 16th days after the insemination. In the first experiment, 413 Holstein-Friesian heifers were used. The cycles of these animals were synchronized with $PGF_2\alpha$ and they were inseminated by observing their estrus. 2.2 mg/kg dose of flunixin meglumine was given to therapy group animals after the insemination's 14th-15th days or 15th-16th days. No application was done to animals in the control group. At the end of this experiment, pregnancy rate in the control group was 58.7% and 58.6% in the treatment group. Serum progesterone levels on 14-15days and 21-22 days after insemination were compared in both pregnant and non-pregnant animals. It was observed that on the 21-22 days progesterone levels of pregnant animals were higher. In the second experiment researchers used 380 Holstein cows and these animals were synchronized by ovsynch protocol. After 16 hours from the second GnRH injection, fixed time artificial insemination was done. 1.4 mg/kg dose of carprofen was given via subcutaneous on the 15th day after the insemination to the treatment group. No therapy was applied to control group. It was identified that while pregnancy rate in carprofen given group was 33%, it was 35.5 in control group. Researchers come to the idea that NSAID application does not affect the reproductive performance.

Heuwieser et al. [72] made a study on 970 cows. They divided the animals into three groups. They administered 1.4 mg/kg dose of carprofen subcutaneous following artificial insemination. 1.4 mg/kg dose of carprofen was given into the uterus 12-24 hours after the insemination to the 2nd group. 3rd group was left as control. After the first insemination the pregnancy rates were found as 42.2%, 38.3% and 45.1%, respectively. As a result they reported that, subcutaneous carprofen therapy did not affect the pregnancy rate but intrauterine therapy had a negative effect on the pregnancy rate.

Amiridis et al. [73] applied flunixin meglumine, ketoprofen and meloxicam to heifers. In the end, they came to conclusion that meloxicam administered animals have the longest estrus cycle and meloxicam is much more potent than other NSAIDs. The same researchers made a study on repeat breeder cows; 1st group was GnRH, 2nd group was progesterone, 3rd group was meloxicam and the 4th group was GnRH + progesterone + meloxicam. They reported that the highest pregnancy rates were seen in 4th group.

In another study on Holstein heifers, 0.5 mg/kg dose of meloxicam was administered subcutaneous on the 15th day following the insemination. Finally, it was identified that pregnancy rate was 24.3% in meloxicam cured group and 52% in control group. In the light of these data, researchers reported that meloxicam application during the time of maternal recognition will be harmful to pregnancy [84].

In a study aimed at increasing pregnancy rate and progesterone synthesis by inhibiting prostaglandin synthesis, a fixed time artificial insemination was done by synchronising cycles of Nelore cows. Researchers divided the animals into 8 groups and they designed the groups as follows. 1st group constitutes the control and given saline on 7th and 16th days; to the 2nd group, saline on the 7th day and flunixin meglumine on the 16th day; to the 3rd group, bST on the 7th day and saline on the 16th day, to the 4th group, bST on the 7th day and flunixin meglumine on the 16th day, to the 5th group, hCG on the 7th day and saline on the 16th day, to the 6th group, hCG on the 7th day and flunixin meglumine on the 16th day, to the 7th group, bST + hCG on the 7th day and saline on the 16th day, to the last group, bST + hCG on the 7th

day and flunixin meglumine on the 16th day were administered. It was found out that the group only cured with hCG on the 7th day showed a higher rate of pregnancy [85].

Tek et al. [86] searched the effects of flunixin meglumine and oxytetracyclin combinations on the cows diagnosed with subclinical endometritis. They applied intramuscular flunixin meglumine (2 mg/kg) and oxytetracyclin (300 mg). They inseminated the animals in the first estrus seen after the application. When compared with the control group, pregnancy rates were higher in flunixin meglumine and oxytetracyclin administered group (25% vs. 55%).

In another study, animals with puerperal metritis were injected with ceftiofur (CEF) and/or flunixin meglumine. CEF was given to the first group for three days. A single dose of flunixin meglumine (2.2 mg/kg) was given intravenous in addition to CEF to the animals in the second group. At the end of the study, researchers came to a conclusion that flunixin meglumine application does not have a beneficial effect on clinical recovery and reproductive performance [87].

13. NSAID use before embryo transfer

Preparing a suitable environment inside uterus is aimed with NSAIDs applied in different times before embryo transfer to cows and heifers. In most of these studies, while flunixin meglumine or ibuprofen applications just before the embryo transfer increase the pregnancy rate has been reported [88-90], in a study it has been reported that it is ineffective [91], and in another study [91] it has been reported that pregnancy rate has diminished.

Elli et al. [88] investigated whether ibuprofen application increases implantation rates during embryo transfer in cattle. In their study done on 100 heifers, they gave half of them 5 mg/kg dose of intramuscular ibuprofen 1 hour before embryo transfer. Pregnancy rate in the treatment group reached 82% but stayed 56% in control group.

Purcell et al. [89], in a study they made on beef cattle applied either 500 mg dose of flunixin meglumine 2-12 minute before embryo transfer or they inserted CIDR shortly after the embryo transfer. The first of four groups was remained as control group, CIDR to 2nd group, flunixin meglumine to 3rd group, both flunixin meglumine given and CIDR inserted to 4th group. Pregnancy rates were found as 65%, 60,7%, 74.7% and 69.8%, respectively. The average pregnancy rates of flunixin meglumine administered animals (3rd and 4th group) and unapplied animals (1st and 2nd group) were identified as 72.3% and 63%.

In another study [90], 10 ml flunixin meglumine was injected to beef cattle 2-5 minutes before the embryo transfer and when it was compared with control group, it was found that pregnancy rate was higher in flunixin meglumine given group (51.1% vs. 63.8%).

McNaughtan [91] injected 10 ml flunixin meglumine to heifers just before the embryo transfer. He identified that during the pregnancy examination 90 days after the embryo transfer, the difference between the therapy and control group (n: 165) was nonsignificant (50% vs. 45%).

Bulbul et al [92] gave 500 mg flunixin meglumine intramuscular five minutes before embryo transfer in a study done on 39 brown Swiss. As a result of the pregnancy examination on the 30th day by means of ultrasound, they reported that pregnancy rate in the flunixin meglumine given group was lower in comparison to control group (50% vs. 52.6%).

14. Conclusions

Artificial insemination is the first biotechnologic application used in domestic animal. It was first performed by Ivanow in 1899 in Russia on farm animals. This procedure was adopted in 1940s by animal breeders and then it has become prominent all over the world. Such associated technologies as cryopreservation, invitro fertilization and embryo transfer have then started to develop and they have resulted in successful pregnancies (93). NSAID implementations have been used in recent years among the assisted reproductive technologies. NSAIDs are applied as a new strategy to increase the pregnancy rates of cows in artificial insemination. Nevertheless, the results obtained from the previous studies conflict with each other. Especially, there are different studies stating that flunixin application increases, does not change or decreases the pregnancy rate. For this reason, NSAIDs relation with interferon tau and endometrial proteins should be investigated in a more detailed way. Thus, from where the difference in pregnancy rates originate can be found and taking of necessary precautions can be possible.

Author details

Zahid Paksoy[1*] and Hüseyin Daş[2]

*Address all correspondence to: paksoyland@yahoo.com, huseyindas@hotmail.com

1 Deparment of Veterinary Sciences, University of Gumushane, Gumushane, Turkey

2 Deparment of Veterinary Sciences, University of Gumushane, Gumushane, Turkey

References

[1] Alaçam E. İnekte İnfertilite Sorunu. In: Alaçam E. (ed.) Evcil Hayvanlarda Doğum ve İnfertilite. İkinci Baskı, Ankara: Medisan Yayınevi; 1999. p267-290.

[2] Çoyan K and Tekeli T. İneklerde Suni Tohumlama. Birinci Baskı, Konya: Bahçıvanlar Basım San. A.Ş.; 1996.

[3] Daşkın A. Sığırcılık İşletmelerinde Reprodüksiyon Yönetimi ve Suni Tohumlama. Ankara: Aydan Web Ofset; 2005.

[4] Gordon I. Reproductive Technology in Farm Animals. Trowbridge: Cromwell Press; 2004.

[5] Noakes ED, Parkinson TJ, England GCW and Arthur GH. Arthur's Veterinary Reproduction and Obstetrics. Eighth Edition, London: Saunders Company; 2001.

[6] Walsh SW, Williams EJ and Evans AC. A review of the causes of poor fertility in high milk producing dairy cows. Animal Reproduction Science 2011;123(3-4) 127-138.

[7] Foote RH. Fertility estimation: a review of past experience and future prospects. Animal Reproduction Science 2003;75(1-2) 119-139.

[8] Al-Makhzoomi A, Lundeheim N, Håård M and Rodríguez-Martínez H. Sperm morphology and fertility of progeny-tested AI dairy bulls in Sweden. Theriogenology 2008;70(4) 682-691.

[9] Saacke RG. Sperm morphology: Its relevance to compensable and uncompensable traits in semen. Theriogenology 2008;70(3) 473-478.

[10] Gillan L, Kroetsch T, Maxwell WM and Evans G. Assessment of in vitro sperm characteristics in relation to fertility in dairy bulls. Animal Reproduction Science 2008;103(3-4) 201-214.

[11] Dinç DA. İneklerde reprodüktif verimliliği artırma programları. Veteriner Hekimler Derneği Dergisi 2006;77(2): 50-64.

[12] Pursley JR, Mee MO and Wiltbank MC. Synchronization of ovulation in dairy cows using PGF2 α and GnRH. Theriogenology 1995;44(7) 915-923.

[13] Santos JEP, Thatcher WW, Chebel RC, Cerri RLA and Galvão KN. The effect of embryonic death rates in cattle on the efficacy of estrus synchronization programs. Animal Reproduction Science 2004;82-83 513-535.

[14] Bozdoğan Ö. Fizyoloji. Ankara: Palme Yayıncılık; 2000.

[15] Paksoy Z and Kalkan C. The effects of GnRH and hCG used during and after artificial insemination on blood serum progesterone levels and pregnancy rate in cows. Kafkas Üniversitesi Veteriner Fakültesi Dergisi 2010;16(3) 371-375.

[16] Binelli M, Thatcher WW, Mattos R and Baruselli PS. Antiluteolytic strategies to improve fertility in cattle. Theriogenology 2001;56(9) 1451-1463.

[17] Rajamahendran R and Sianangama PC. Effect of human chorionic gonadotrophin on dominant follicles in cows: formation of accessory corpora lutea, progesterone production and pregnancy rates. Journal of Reproduction and Fertility 1992;95 577-584.

[18] Santos JEP, Thatcher WW, Pool L and Overton MW. Effect of human chorionic gonadotropin on luteal function and reproductive performance of high-producing holstein dairy cows. Journal of Animal Science 2001;79 2881-2894.

[19] Kharche SD and Srivastava SK. Dose dependent effect of GnRH analogue on pregnancy rate of repeat breeder crossbred cows. Animal Reproduction Science 2007;99 196–201.

[20] Sheldon IM and Dobson H. Effect of gonadotrophin releasing hormone administered 11 days after insemination on the pregnancy rates of cattle to the first and later services. Veterinary Record 1993;133 160-163.

[21] Ullah G, Fuquay JW, Keawkhong T, Clark BL, Pogue DE and Murpheys EJ. Effect of Gonadotropin-releasing hormone at estrus on subsequent luteal function and fertility in lactating holsteins during heat stress. Journal Dairy Science 1996;79(11) 1950-1953.

[22] Kalkan C and Horoz H. Pubertas ve Seksüel Sikluslar. In: Alaçam E. (ed.) Evcil Hayvanlarda Doğum ve İnfertilite. Ankara: Medisan Yayınevi; 1997. p13-30.

[23] Clarke IJ and Pompolo S. Synthesis and secretion of GnRH. Animal Reproduction Science 2005;88(1-2) 29-55.

[24] Hopkins SM. Reproductive Patterns of Cattle. In: Pineada MH (ed.) McDonald's Veterinary Endocrinology and Reproduction. Fifth Edition, Iowa: Iowa State Press; 2003. p395-411.

[25] Ball PJH and Peters AR. Reproduction in Cattle. Third Edition, Oxford: Blackwell Publishing; 2004.

[26] Guyton AC and Hall JE., editors. Introduction to Endocrinology - Textbook of Medical Physiology, Eleventh Edition, Philadelphia: Elsevier Saunders; 2006.

[27] Hassa O and Aştı RN. Embriyoloji. Ankara: Yorum Basın Yayın Sanayi Ltd; 1997.

[28] Ulukaya E. Steroid Hormonlar. In: Tokullugil A, Dirican M and Ulukaya E (eds.) Biyokimya. İstanbul: Nobel Tıp Kitabevleri; 1997.

[29] Aktümsek A. Anatomi ve Fizyoloji. Ankara: Nobel Yayın Dağıtım; 2001.

[30] Lawrence TLJ and Fowler VR. Growth of Farm Animals. Second Edition, Trowbridge: Cromwell Press; 2002.

[31] Özden M. Anatomi ve Fizyoloji. Ankara: Kadıoğlu Matbaası; 1990.

[32] Senger PL. Pathways to Pregnancy and Parturition. Second Edition, Pullman: Current Conception, Inc.; 2003.

[33] Hansen TR, Austin KJ, Perry DJ, Pru JK, Teixeira MG and Johnson GA. Mechanism of action of interferon-tau in the uterus during early pregnancy. J Reprod Fertil Suppl 1999;54 329-339.

[34] Vassilev N, Yotov S and Dimitrov F. Incidence of early embryonic death in dairy cows. Trakia Journal of Sciences 2005;3(5) 62-64.

[35] Bartolome JA, Kamimura S, Silvestre F, Arteche ACM, Trigg T and Thatcher WW. The use of a deslorelin implant (GnRH agonist) during the late embryonic period to reduce pregnancy loss. Theriogenology 2006;65 1443–1453.

[36] Inskeep EK. Preovulatory, postovulatory, and postmaternal recognition effects of concentrations of progesterone on embryonic survival in the cow. Journal of Animal Science 2004;82 E24-39.

[37] Ahmad N, Schrick FN, Butcher RL and Inskeep EK. Effect of persistent follicles on early embryonic losses in beef cows. Biology of Reproduction 1995;52 1129-1135.

[38] Wolfenson D, Roth Z and Meidan R. Impaired reproduction in heat-stressed cattle: basic and applied aspects. Animal Reproduction Science 2000;60-61 535-547.

[39] Hafez ESE, Jainudeen MR and Rosnina Y. Hormones, Growth Factors, and Reproduction. In: Hafez B and Hafez ESE (eds) Reproduction in Farm Animals. Seventh Edition, Philadelphia: Lippincott Williams & Wilkins; 2000. p33-54.

[40] Morrow DA. Current Therapy in Theriogenology 2. Philadelphia: WB Saunders Company; 1986.

[41] Hasçelik Z. Nonsteroid Antiinflamatuvar ilaçlar, Sürekli Tıp Eğitimi Dergisi 2001;10,1.

[42] Saraf S. NSAIDs: Non-steroidal Anti-Inflammatory Drugs: An Overview, PharmaMed Press. 2008.

[43] Salman MC, Özyüncü Ö, Aksu T and Günalp S. Jinekolojide Cox-2 inhibitörlerinin kullanımı, Hacettepe Tıp Dergisi 2004;35 65-68.

[44] Botting RM. Cyclooxygenase: Past, present and future. A tribute to John R. Vane (1927–2004), Journal of Thermal Biology 2006;31(1-2) 208-219.

[45] Rao P and Knaus EE. Evolution of nonsteroidal anti-inflammatory drugs (NSAIDs): cyclooxygenase (COX) inhibition and beyond. J Pharm Pharm Sci 2008;11(2) 81-110.

[46] Myers R. The Basics of Chemistry. Greenwood Publishing Group; 2003.

[47] Isakson PC. Pharmacology of Cox-2 inhibitors, In: Dannenberg AJ and DuBois RN (eds.) Cox-2: a new target for cancer prevention and treatment. Basel, Switzerland; 2003. p25-51.

[48] Chandrasekharan NV, Dai H, Roos KL, Evanson NK, Tomsik J, Elton TS and Simmons DL. COX-3, a cyclooxygenase-1 variant inhibited by acetaminophen and other analgesic /antipyretic drugs: cloning, structure, and expression. PNAS 2002;99,21 13926-13931.

[49] Divers TJ. COX Inhibitors: Making the Best Choice for the Laminitic case, Journal of Equine Veterinary Science 2008; 28(6) 367-369,

[50] Salhab AS, Gharaibeh MN, Shomaf MS and Amro BI. Meloxicam inhibits rabbit ovulation. Contraception 2001;63 329–333.

[51] Salhab AS, Amro BI and Shomaf MS. Further investigation on meloxicam contraceptivity in female rabbits: luteinizing unruptured follicles, a microscopic evidence. Contraception 2003;67 485–489.

[52] Shafiq N, Malhotra S and Pandhi P. Comparison of nonselective cyclo-oxygenase (COX) inhibitor and selective COX-2 inhibitors on preimplantation loss, postimplantation loss and duration of gestation: an experimental study. Contraception 2004;69 71-75.

[53] Gaytán M, Bellido C, Morales C, Sánchez-Criado JE and Gaytán F. Effects of selective inhibition of cyclooxygenase and lipooxygenase pathways in follicle rupture and ovulation in the rat, Reproduction 2006;132 571-577.

[54] Poyser NL. A comparison of the effects of indomethacin and NS-398 (a selective prostaglandin H synthase-2 inhibitor) on implantation in the rat, Prostaglandins, Leukotrienes and Essential Fatty Acids 1999;61,5 297-301.

[55] Bukowski R, Mackay L, Fittkow C, Shi L, Saade GR and Garfield RE. Inhibition of cervical ripening by local application of cyclooxygenase 2 inhibitor, American Journal of Obstetrics & Gynecology 2001;184(7) 1374-1379.

[56] Muzii L, Marana R, Brunetti L, Margutti F, Vacca M and Mancuso S. Postoperative adhesion prevention with low-dose aspirin: effect through the selective inhibition of thromboxane production. Human Reproduction 1998;13(6) 1486-1489.

[57] Slattery MM, Friel AM, Healy DG and Morrison JJ. Uterine Relaxant Effects of Cyclooxygenase-2 Inhibitors In Vitro. Obstetrics & Gynecology 2001;98(4) 563-569.

[58] Guvenal T, Cetin A, Ozdemir H, Yanar O and Kaya T. Prevention of postoperative adhesion formation in rat uterine horn model by nimesulide: a selective COX-2 inhibitor. Human Reproduction 2001;16(8) 1732-1735.

[59] Reese J, Brown N, Paria BC, Morrow J and Dey SK. COX-2 compensation in the uterus of COX-1 deficient mice during the pre-implantation period. Molecular and Cellular Endocrinology 1999;150, 23-31.

[60] Chakraborty I, Das SK, Wang J and Dey SK. Developmental expression of the cyclooxygenase-1 and cyclo-oxygenase-2 genes in the peri-implantation mouse uterus and their differential regulation by the blastocyst and ovarian steroids. Journal of Molecular Endocrinology 1996;16 107-122,

[61] Lim H, Paria BC, Das SK, Dinchuk JE, Langenbach R, Trzaskos JM and Dey SK. Multiple Female Reproductive Failures in Cyclooxygenase 2–Deficient Mice. Cell 1997;91 197-208.

[62] Boothe DM. The Analgesic, Antipyretic, Anti-inflammatory Drugs. In: Veterinary pharmacology and therapeutics, Ed: Adams HR. Eighth edition, Blackwell Publishing, Iowa, 2001. p433.

[63] Scott PR, Penny CD and McCrae AI. Cattle Medicine. Manson Publishing, London, UK. 2011.

[64] Braun W. Periparturient Infections and Structural Abnormalities. In: Youngquist RS, Threlfall WR. (eds.) Current Therapy In Large Animal Theriogenology, Second Edition, Saunders Company, 2007. p573.

[65] Radostits OM, Gay CC, Hinchcliff KW and Constable PD. Veterinary Medicine, A textbook of the diseases of cattle, horses, sheep, pigs and goats. Tenth edition, Saunders Company, 2006. p58-59.

[66] Woolums AR, Baker JC and Smith JA. Upper respiratory tract Diseases. In: Large Animal Internal Medicine, Ed: Smith BP. Fourth edition, Mosby Company, 2009. p592.

[67] Blikslager AT and Jones SL. Disorders of the Esophagus. In: Smith BP (ed.) Large Animal Internal Medicine. Fourth edition, Mosby Company, 2009. p690.

[68] Mackay RJ. Endotoxemia. In: Smith BP (ed.) Large Animal Internal Medicine. Fourth edition, Mosby Company, 2009. p722.

[69] Jones SL. Medical Disorders of the Large Intestine. In: Smith BP (ed.) Large Animal Internal Medicine. Fourth edition, Mosby Company, 2009. p749.

[70] Romich JA. Fundamentals of Pharmacology for Veterinary Technicians, Second Edition, Delmar, Cengage Learning. 2010.

[71] Plumb DC. Plumb's Veterinary Drug Handbook, 7th Edition. PharmaVet Inc. 2011.

[72] Heuwieser W, Iwersen M and Goetze L. Efficacy of carprofen on conception rates in lactating dairy cows after subcutaneous or intrauterine administration at the time of breeding. Journal of Dairy Science 2011;94(1) 146-151.

[73] Amiridis GS, Tsiligianni T, Dovolou E, Rekkas C, Vouzaras D and Menegatos I. Combined administration of gonadotropin-releasing hormone, progesterone, and meloxicam is an effective treatment for the repeat-breeder cow. Theriogenology 2009;72(4) 542-548.

[74] Guzeloglu A, Erdem H, Saribay MK, Thatcher WW and Tekeli T. Effect of the administration of flunixin meglumine on pregnancy rates in Holstein heifers. Veterinary Record 2007;160(12) 404-406.

[75] Merrill ML, Ansotegui RP, Wamsley NE, Burns PD and Geary TW. Effects of Flunixin Meglumine on Embryonic Loss in Stressed Beef Cows. Proceedings, Western Section, American Society of Animal Science; 2003.

[76] Merrill ML, Ansotegui RP, Paterson JA, and Geary TW. Effect of Flunixin Meglumine on Early Embryonic Mortality in Stressed Beef Females. Proceedings, Western Section, American Society of Animal Science 2004;55 304-307.

[77] Merrill ML, Ansotegui RP, Burns PD, MacNeil MD and Geary TW. Effects of flunixin meglumine and transportation on establishment of pregnancy in beef cows. Journal of Animal Science 2007;85(6) 1547-1554.

[78] Lucacin E, Pinto-Neto A, Mota MF, Acco A, Souza MIL, Alberton J and Silva AV. Effects of flunixin meglumine on reproductive parameters in beef cattle. Anim. Reprod. 2010;7(2) 75-79.

[79] Rabaglino MB, Risco CA, Thatcher MJ, Lima F, Santos JE and Thatcher WW. Use of a five-day progesterone-based timed AI protocol to determine if flunixin meglumine improves pregnancy per timed AI in dairy heifers. Theriogenology 2010;73(9) 1311-1318.

[80] Geary TW, Ansotegui RP, MacNeil MD, Roberts AJ and Waterman RC. Effects of flunixin meglumine on pregnancy establishment in beef cattle. Journal of Animal Science 2010;88(3) 943-949.

[81] Odensvik K, Gustafsson H and Kindahl H. The effect on luteolysis by intensive oral administration of flunixin granules in heifers. Animal Reproduction Science 1998;50(1-2) 35-44.

[82] Doğruer G, Sarıbay MK and Karaca F. Repeat Breeder Sorunlu Düvelerde Fluniksin Meglumin Uygulamalarının Gebelik Oranı Üzerine Etkisi. Fırat Üniversitesi Sağlık Bilimleri dergisi 2007;21(6) 263-268.

[83] von Krueger X and Heuwieser W. Effect of flunixin meglumine and carprofen on pregnancy rates in dairy cattle. Journal of Dairy Science 2010;93(11) 5140-5146.

[84] Erdem H and Guzeloglu A. Effect of meloxicam treatment during early pregnancy in Holstein heifers. Reproduction in Domestic Animals 2010;45(4) 625-628.

[85] Rossetti RC, Perdigão A, Mesquita FS, Sá Filho M, Nogueira GP, Machado R, Membrive CM and Binelli M. Effects of flunixin meglumine, recombinant bovine somatotropin and/or human chorionic gonadotropin on pregnancy rates in Nelore cows. Theriogenology 2011;76(4) 751-758.

[86] Tek Ç, Sabuncu A, İkiz S, Bağcıgil F, Gündüz MC, Kılıçarslan MR and Özgür Y. The effect of a single administration of parenteral oxytetracycline and flunixin meglumine combination on the reproductive performance of dairy cows with subclinical endometritis. Turkish Journal of Veterinary and Animal Sciences. 2010;34(4) 319-325.

[87] Drillich M, Voigt D, Forderung D and Heuwieser W. Treatment of acute puerperal metritis with flunixin meglumine in addition to antibiotic treatment. Journal of Dairy Science 2007;90(8) 3758-3763.

[88] Elli M, Gaffuri B, Frigerio A, Zanardelli M, Covini D, Candiani M and Vignali M. Effect of a single dose of ibuprofen lysinate before embryo transfer on pregnancy rates in cows. Reproduction 2001;121(1) 151-154.

[89] Purcell SH, Beal WE and Gray KR. Effect of a CIDR insert and flunixin meglumine, administered at the time of embryo transfer, on pregnancy rate and resynchronization of estrus in beef cattle. Theriogenology 2005;64(4) 867-878.

[90] Schrick FN, Hockett ME, Towns TM, Saxton AM, Wert NE and Wehrman ME. Administration of a Prostaglandin Inhibitor Immediately Prior to Embryo Transfer Improves Pregnancy Rates in Cattle. Theriogenology 2001;55 370 (Abstract).

[91] McNaughtan J. The Effect of Prostaglandin Inhibitor on Pregnancy Rates of Heifer Embryo Transfer Recipients. Master Thesis, Brigham Young University Utah; 2004.

[92] Bülbül B, Dursun S, Kırbas M, Köse M and Ümütlü S. The Effect of Flunixin Meglumine Injected Before Embryo Transfer on Pregnancy Rates in Heifers. Kafkas Universitesi Veteriner Fakültesi Dergisi 2010,16(1) 105-109.

[93] Foote RH. The history of artificial insemination: Selected notes and notables. Journal of Animal Science 2002;80 1-10.

Chapter 6

Molecular Markers in Sperm Analysis

Rita Payan-Carreira, Paulo Borges,
Fernando Mir and Alain Fontbonne

Additional information is available at the end of the chapter

http://dx.doi.org/10.5772/52231

1. Introduction

In mammals, the success of fertilization largely depends on gamete fertility potential and consequently on what concerns sperm and oocyte quality they are both equally important.

Sperm contribution to fertilization is usually estimated through evaluation of semen parameters. A loss of fertility potential associated to manipulation and preservation techniques is usually calculated based on the semen characteristics at collection and on the knowledge of the damages associated with the technique to be implemented.

Assessment of sperm quality conventionally relies on microscopic evaluation of sperm parameters including total sperm count, sperm concentration, percentage of motile sperm and percentage of normal sperm morphology. Some of these parameters are correlated with fertility though it does not truthfully predict male fertility [1-3]. Concentration and morphology are considered to be important to evaluate the fertilizing ability of sperm cells, as well as motility and the acrosome status, which are critical elements regarding fertilization. These parameters are currently analysed under light microscopy. Computer-assisted semen analysis (CASA) increases the reliability and the accuracy of the analysis with the increase of cell counting [4,5]. Results of the functional testing (such as the *zona pellucida* binding assay, the hemi-zona essay or the hypoosmotic swelling test) are better correlated with the AI outcome than the results of conventional semen evaluation [1,2].

Nevertheless, these methods have limited prognostic value for the reproductive success of the donor male [6,7]. Discrete and unclear sperm abnormalities impairing the reproductive success of sperm and egg interaction often remain undiagnosed. This is the major limitation for the most conservational *in vitro* methodologies of sperm evaluation, either in humans or animals. Inability of the *in vitro* assessment methods to accurately predict spermatozoa fertility may be attributed to the complexity and multifactorial nature of male fertility.

In the past decades, attempts to escape these limits led to the introduction, in the laboratorial panel, of some sophisticated analyses. Those included the use of fluorescent markers to assess the acrosomal status, the use of vital staining for mitochondrial activity, the use of particular fluorochromes to detect altered sperm chromatin or DNA integrity along with several molecular regulators of thermal and oxidative stress. Proteomic, biochemical, and immunocytochemical approaches are now starting to highlight some key events that may determine the success of the sperm function. Existing functional tests were also retained, such as the hypoosmotic swelling test and the hemi-zone assay, to assess membrane functional integrity and sperm ability to interplay with the oocyte.

Understanding the main determinants of sperm fertility and knowing how fertility changes or is influenced by sperm manipulation (such as cryopreservation and sperm-sorting) would allow to enhance the knowledge on extender design, to accurately estimate sperm fertility and to predict sperm survival after processing. The knowledge to adequately extend the lifespan of cryopreserved sperm would also be improved, in particular on what concerns the programs for genetic biodiversity preservation. Nowadays, the lack of reliable methods allowing the accurate *in vitro* assessment of semen quality, limits our capacity to properly monitor semen freezing-thawing damages and to predict its performance at insemination [8].

Though extensively used in domestic species (such as bovine, pigs and dogs), it is well known and accepted that cryopreservation damages the sperm, with a large number of cells losing their fertility potential after freezing/thawing. Further, it is also common knowledge that individual variations exist on sperm resistance to cell damage during these procedures, justifying why some males are "better freezers" than others, even if no differences are found in fresh semen quality assessment [9, 10].

Determination of additional markers for semen quality is now being explored either as a complementary assessment of sperm quality or as an additional way to study in more detail the side effects of extenders or molecules associated to infertility. Seminal markers reveal molecular pathways that could be suppressed or stimulated by *in vitro* sperm manipulation. Moreover, it may be of utmost importance when considering the development of protocols for sperm cryopreservation of wild and endangered species. Up to now, the extender selection in those species is mainly based on phylogenetic or physiological resemblances and on the trial-and-error approach.

Another issue strengthening the need for additional tests in laboratory assessment of sperm quality relates to the fact that standard seminal parameters (motility, concentration and morphology) currently used for all the species are insufficient to predict fertility and to detect sub-fertile males. In addition, sperm samples are very heterogeneous and although spermatozoa may look the same on traditional semen analysis, more sophisticated methods allow identifying different spermatozoa subpopulations with distinct biochemical and physiological characteristics. It is the combination of sperm cells of different functional competences that largely determines the fertility potential of a specific male.

http://dx.doi.org/10.5772/52231

The search for effective predictors of spermatozoa fertility is now on the table, and the identification of suitable molecules would greatly benefit the semen industry and would strengthen the proposal of new therapies for infertility, in both man and animal. Furthermore, it would allow a better understanding of the side effects of technology (such as freezing/thawing or sex-sorting procedures) upon the sperm integrity and functionality, as well as to evaluate the reasons of some undesirable responses of exotic or endangered species' sperm to preservation.

A large number of factors and molecules have been proposed to be of interest or tested as putative predictors for sperm fertility. Before playing their role in fertilization, spermatozoa are required to survive in the female genitalia, accomplish to reach the place for fertilization and to acquire competence to fertilize the oocyte (Figure 1). This is true, for both the natural mating and the artificial insemination. These are important actions, which reflect a multitude of complex and specialised functions that, in brief, result in sperm survival and fertility. Yet, all these functions would hardly be evaluated together through a sole molecule.

In this review it is the intent to present and discuss the use of new methods for sperm assessment and estimation of spermatozoa fertility.

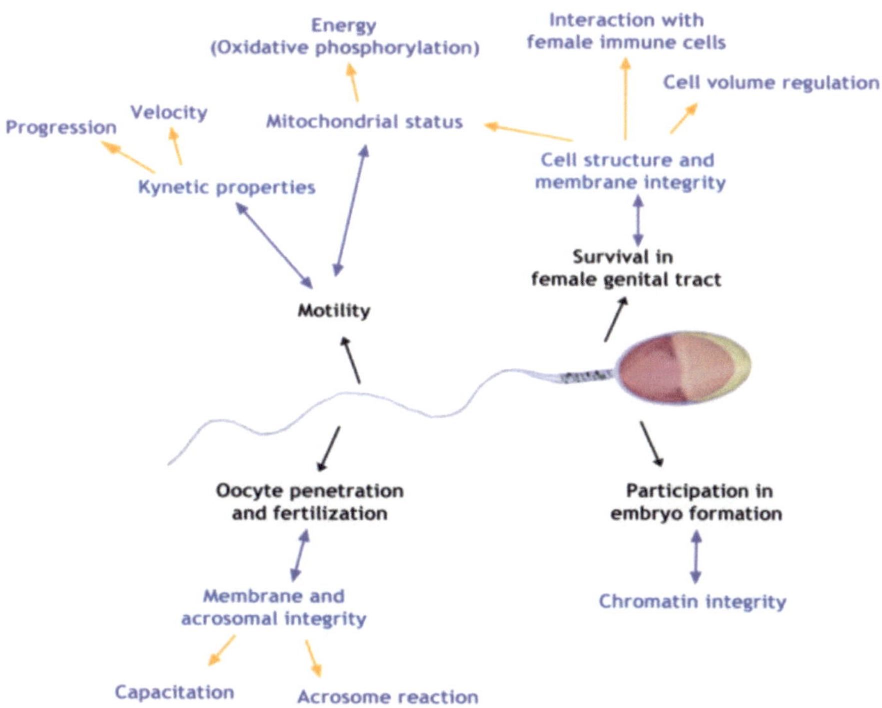

Figure 1. Major cellular mechanisms associated with main roles of the spermatozoon.

2. Proposed side effects for sperm cryopreservation

Sperm cryopreservation is unavoidably linked to a reduction in sperm quality, which has been related to cold shock and freezing damages. The importance of cold shock injuries varies with the species, the composition of the extender, the cryoprotectant selected and the male, among other factors [10,11]. Seldom more than 50% of the sperm population survives cryopreservation [9].

Deleterious effects of freezing/thawing procedures originate a reduction on the sperm life span due to alterations in the structure and functions of spermatozoa. Side effects include altered motility, changes in the plasma membrane and acrosomal integrity and increased DNA fragmentation. All these alterations induce a reduction of the sperm ability to survive in the female reproductive tract and to interact with the oocyte at fertilization [8,12]. In an attempt to compensate these side effects, seminal doses are usually prepared with excessive numbers of spermatozoa in order to improve AI fertility [5,8].

Available cryopreservation techniques have a number of potentially detrimental problems, such as physical and chemical injuries that prone the spermatozoa to cell death and dysfunction (Figure 2). These include [9,13-15]:

- Capacitation-like changes – after freezing/thawing, sperm behaves as if capacitated, which decreases its ability to survive within the female genital tract and to fuse with the oocyte;
- Motility impairment – a decrease in the motility is observed in post-thawed spermatozoa, which tend to exhibit a variable degree of motility weakening, with subsequent hampering of sperm progression till the oviducts and a decrease on the fertility potential;
- Oxidative damages – which may trigger apoptosis and DNA damage when reaching a given threshold. Apoptosis compromises the mitochondrial function, motility and predispose to DNA fragmentation.
- Compromise of the membrane and acrosome integrity - loss of membrane integrity lead to altered ionic transport to the cell, in particular the calcium and water balance, with subsequent loss of the sperm ability for volume regulation and osmoadaptation. Also, it will compromise protein location and/or exposition on the cell's surface, which negatively affects sperm survival, sperm binding to oviductal epithelium and interaction between male and female gametes. In addition, restrain of the acrosome integrity may compromise sperm competence to penetrate the oocyte layers at fertilization;
- DNA and chromatin changes, which may not be directly related to fertilization but are often reported to impair sustainable post-syngamy embryonic development and pregnancy.

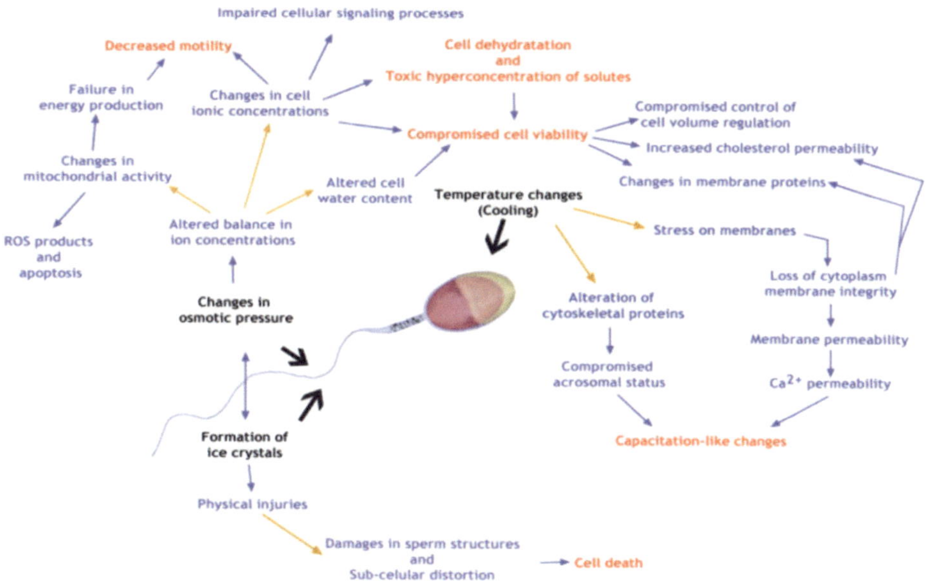

Figure 2. Proposed deleterious effects in sperm cryopreservation [Ca^{2+} - calcium].

3. Biological markers of sperm function

The most frequently used methods of sperm analysis have been pleasantly reviewed in a recent InTech publication [11], driving the main topic of this review into new adjunctive methods available to test sperm quality (Figure 3). These tests can be performed as well in freshly ejaculated sperm or in preserved samples. In the former, it would allow to increase the ability to predict sperm quality, the selection of donor/sperm for cryopreservation and to assess infertility causes. In the later it could be of utmost interest to study the sperm response to preservation trials, such as the design of a new extender. Further, it could also be of importance when studying the sperm response to preservation in new species, where it would allow the identification of the most suitable molecular and functionally-friendly extender or procedure.

3.1. Assessment of events associated with sperm capacitation

For long, it has been accepted that freezing/thawing procedures induce a capacitation-like status that originate losses on the fertilizing potential of spermatozoa. Non-capacitated live sperm cells survive longer in the female genital tract than capacitated sperm [16]. Dysfunction of intracellular pathways associated with calcium (Ca^{2+}) predisposes to acrosome instability and exocytosis of its content. Regulation of protein function by Ca^{2+} signalling pathways is central for most sperm functions and infertility is often found when those signalling pathways are disturbed [17].

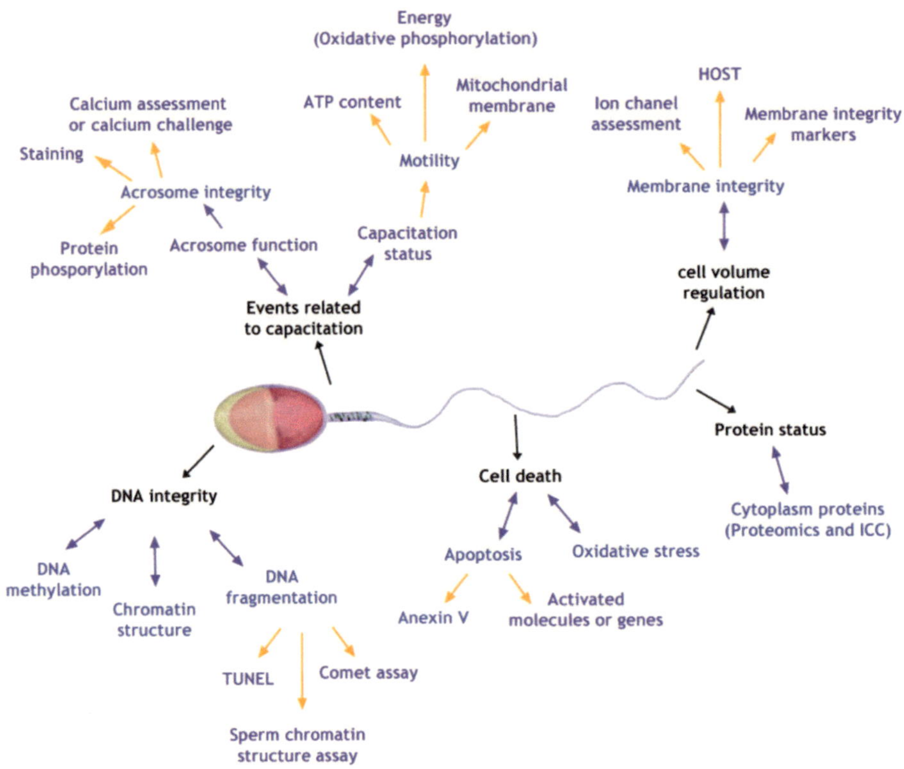

Figure 3. Main objectives for advanced sperm screening are directly related to the assessment of the spermatozoa functions [ICC - immunocytochemistry; HOST - hypoosmotic swelling test; TUNEL - Terminal deoxynucleotidyl transferase dUTP nick end labeling].

As it was mentioned, calcium is an important regulator of intracellular activity. Calcium mobilization has been associated with major sperm functions, such as capacitation, acrosome reaction and hypermotility. Ca^{2+} stores in the sperm are located in the acrosome, neck and mitochondria [17]. Release of Ca^{2+} from its stores triggers the above-mentioned reactions, although it is now suspected that different patterns of calcium release are responsible for different functions. For example, hypermotility is associated with an oscillatory, wave-like pattern of Ca^{2+} release, while capacitation, acrosome reaction and exocytosis of the content are associated with a burst of intracellular Ca^{2+} into the cytoplasm [6,17]. Also, the increase in free intracellular Ca^{2+} is often associated with the stimulation of different, pH-sensitive ion-channels that have been associated with hypermotility and acrosome reaction. Sperm neck Ca^{2+} stores seem to be related with the flagella movement, during hyperactivation [17].

Acrosome membrane integrity is commonly assessed with fluorescent conjugated lectins (PNA- Peanut agglutinin- and PSA- Pisum sativum agglutinin). Absence of fluorescence in the living sperm indicates an intact acrosome, whilst fluorescence is indicative of acrosome disrupted or acrosome-reacted sperm [5,11]. Fluorescent conjugated lectins can be used either in flow cytometry [18] or in cell imaging microscopy, and when combined with other vital staining, such as Hoechst 33258 or 33342 and carboxy-SNARF/PI (carboxy-seminaphthorhodafluor/ propidium iodide), or with the hypoosmotic swelling test they also allow to distinguish between non-viable and reacted spermatozoa.

There are other fluorescent tests to evaluate the acrosome, like the chlortetracyclin (CTC) staining, in which fluorescence is activated when there is bounding to free calcium ions. When combined with another fluorescent dye, such as Hoechst 33258, the combined fluorescent staining allows to differentiate from three different sperm populations: the uncapacitated and acrosome intact (F-pattern), the capacitated and acrosome intact (B-pattern) and the capacitated and acrosome reacted (AR-pattern) [5]. Today, CTC staining is a routine test to assess the occurrence of the capacitation and the acrosome reaction; it has also been adapted to flow cytometry analysis.

Additional tests can be performed for assessment of the occurrence of capacitation-like events, using biological markers, molecules known to trigger or participate in the capacitation reaction. Determining the cholesterol efflux, the protein phosphorylation and changes in intracellular calcium are some of the available methodologies. Nevertheless, for some indicators, it is still unclear how they correlate with sperm quality.

Furthermore, the acrosome status may be tested indirectly through calcium assessment or by studying the response of sperm stimulation with calcium ionophores, progesterone or egg vestments [14,15,17,19]. Acrosome defective sperm show poorer responses to calcium testing than do the sperm with intact acrosome [6].

Changes in free Ca^{2+} concentrations in sperm may be studied by flow cytometry or indirectly by an ionophore challenge test, the later generating intracellular calcium signals that trigger the acrosome reaction [14,15,20]. The percentage of reacted spermatozoa is usually determined using a fluorescent dye. Samples with 10 to 30% of reacted spermatozoa have higher fertility potential than samples with less than 10% (this value being considered a threshold) [20].

Recently, it was demonstrated that sperm exposition to progesterone induced similar but more rapid Ca^{2+} signalling pathway, which seems to be independent of a known second messenger system [19]. This behaviour allows the use of this molecule to challenge the sperm acrosome function, as do the ionophore test. For a large number of species, granulosa cells expelled with the oocyte from the ovulatory follicle have the capacity to produce progesterone, which can affect the spermatozoa that approaches the egg for fertilization.

Protein phosphorylation can be studied using different approaches. Detection of phosphotyrosine residues in the spermatozoa can be performed by immunocytochemistry (ICC) in a cytology specimen (over silane- or poly-L-lysine-coated slides), using specific antibodies. The reaction is amplified by the use of secondary antibodies and the reaction may be visualized either with a fluorescent or a non-fluorescent dye. Further, this technique also allows the assessment of sub-cellular changes in the molecule localisation, besides the evaluation of changes in the intensity of immunolabelling [7]. ICC may also extend to other proteins targeting acrosome-related functions.

While ICC locates the molecule inside the cell, the Western blotting technique (also named immunoblotting) may be used for quantification of the protein. After a gel electrophoresis, the extracted proteins are transposed into a membrane and incubated with a primary antibody for the target molecule (the same as for ICC). The reaction is revealed in an X-ray film or a digital image [21]. The use of a cell or a molecular standard, like for the genomic assays, will allow the relative quantification of the protein content in the sample. However, this technique presents a weakness: the possible degradation of the target protein during sample preparation may cause the visualization of multiple bands of different molecular weight.

Mass spectrometry and liquid chromatography, enhancing the separation and the identification of a large number of proteins, are often used for proteomics analysis. However, until now, this method gives a catalogue of hundreds or thousands of proteins that are not easily associated with sperm biological functions [22,23] and consequently there is not a practical interest for the immediate sperm quality assessment. Yet, using specific regions of spermatozoa or particular cell organelles to focus the analysis could turn this approach to be helpful in the assessment of sperm function or specific sperm events.

3.2. Assessment of energy metabolism and sperm motility

Energy metabolism is a key-factor in sperm function. It is supported by ATP pathway, which is found in the background of the most important sperm events, such as hyperactivation, capacitation and protein phosphorylation of the acrosome reaction. It has been shown that high intracellular ATP values correlate with higher survival and vitality post-freezing/thawing [24], while mitochondrial membrane potential mirrors the sperm quality and a better motility pattern. A primary function associated with mitochondria is the ATP synthesis by oxidative phosphorylation, although, energy might also be obtained by glycogenolysis in the sperm tail, a necessary complement to sustain energy in the tail and to maintain an effective movement. In humans, a decrease in mitochondrial activity has been found in patients with history of infertility even when normozoospermic [25]. Also, cumulative evidences suggest that mitochondrial activity is positively correlated with sperm quality and fertility, possibly associated with the fact that healthy mitochondria have a higher membrane potential [25].

The intracellular ATP content may be determined by an enzymatic assay (ATP/NADH-linked enzyme coupling assay) in association with spectrophotometry. On this reaction, the regeneration of hydrolysed ATP is linked to NADH oxidation. The assay measures the differences in NADH, which are proportional to the rate of ATP hydrolysis.

Sperm metabolic function may also be evaluated by assessment of the mitochondrial activity. Integrity of the mitochondrial functioning can be assessed using specific dyes for these organelles [7,43]. Earlier, rhodamine 123 (R123) was frequently used to selectively stain functional mitochondria. It is a potentiometric membrane dye that fluoresces only when the proton gradient over the inner mitochondrial membrane (IMM) is built up. When the proton gradient collapses, the aerobic production of ATP fails, and mitochondria remain unstained [13]. More recently, other dyes have been developed, which selectively bind to respirating mitochondria and become fluorescent after oxidation. These can be used to test mitochondrial functionality, which has been correlated with the mitochondrial potential [25]. They are named MitoTracker® and are available in red, green and orange colours. Live sperm cells are suspended to incubate into a solution with the selected probe. Cells may be analysed by flow cytometry, by microplate-based analysis or by epifluorescence microscopy, using cytological preparations. The probes diffuse across the plasma membrane and accumulate in active mitochondria. To determine the percentage of MitoTracker positive sperm, 200 spermatozoa are usually counted per sample, in at least four fields, in a fluorescence microscope [7], varying the spectral wavelength with the probe used. The MitoTracker® can be combined with a vital dye, such as the Hoechst 33342, allowing the separation of different sperm sub-populations: the dead spermatozoa, the live mitochondrial non-competent sperm and the live mitochondrial competent spermatozoa. Also belonging to the MitoTracker dyes, JC-1 (5,5',6,6'-tetrachloro-1,1',3,3'- tetraethylbenzimidazolylcarbocyanine iodide) is a dual-emission, potential-sensitive probe, which emits different fluorescent colours according to the membrane potential (IMM): after incubation JC-1 is captured by functional mitochondria where it stains in green if the IMM is polarized or in orange or red if the IMM is depolarized. Depolarization of IMM leads to the aggregation of the dye. The ratio of orange-to-green JC-1 fluorescence depends only on the membrane potential, since it is independent of the mitochondrial size, shape or density. Using this staining, a sperm sample can be composed of different combinations of fluorescent cells according to their mitochondrial inner membrane potential [13]. The different labelling patterns may be correlated with parameters such as sperm motility [7].

A different approach to assess the mitochondrial integrity is to assess the presence of sperm mitochondrial proteins through the use of ICC [7,13]. This approach allows the detection and location of target molecules within the cell and the study of the modifications to the expected pattern of immunolabelling. One of the proteins available to study mitochondrial function is the Cytochrome C oxidase or complex IV, which catalyzes the final step in the mitochondrial electron transfer chain. This molecule is regarded as one of the major regulatory molecules for oxidative phosphorylation. As in other ICC, cytological preparations are set to incubate with the specific primary antibody, followed by incubation with the appropriated secondary antibody. The revelation can be obtained with DAB (3,3-Diaminobenzidine) or using DAPI (4',6-diamidino-2-phenylindole) as fluorochrome, under light or epifluorescence microscopy, respectively. The percentage of stained cells is determined over 200 spermatozoa in a minimum of 4 microscope fields.

Heat Shock Proteins (HSP), which are divided in families, are chaperon proteins involved in the protection of intracellular macromolecules against unfolding and aggregation during thermal and osmotic stress. HSP70 and HSP90, which have been found in the sperm, have important functions in the cellular trafficking of proteins other than the refolding and transport of client proteins. The role of HSP's on cell signalling in mature sperm is not clearly understood. It is known that an active cell metabolism, such as ATP production, is required for the expression of heat sock response [26,27]. HSP 70 and HSP 90 have separated ATPase and client protein-binding sites [27] and also distinct roles in sperm function. It has been shown that HSP70 and 90 are targets for protein phosphorylation, which is activated during capacitation and capacitation-like response to sperm manipulation, in a reaction that might be associated with the nitric oxide synthesis during oxidative stress [28]. Sperm is transcriptionally inactive. Thus, HSP content in the spermatozoa is defined at ejaculation and those proteins must be present in the cytosol to help protecting the sperm from injury [29]. Therefore it is expectable to find a reduction of its amount or intensity of immunoexpression for these molecules (if Western blotting or ICC were used) after the cell attack. In canine ejaculates, a diminished number of sperm cells with low immunoreaction for HSP70 was found in semen of good quality. A reduction of the intensity of immunolabelling for this molecule was found after freezing/thawing (Figure 4), along with dislocation of the immunostaining from the acrosomal area to the sperm tail [30,31]. It has also been found a correlation between HSP70 immunoreaction in freshly ejaculated sperm and sperm damage after freezing/thawing procedures [30,31].

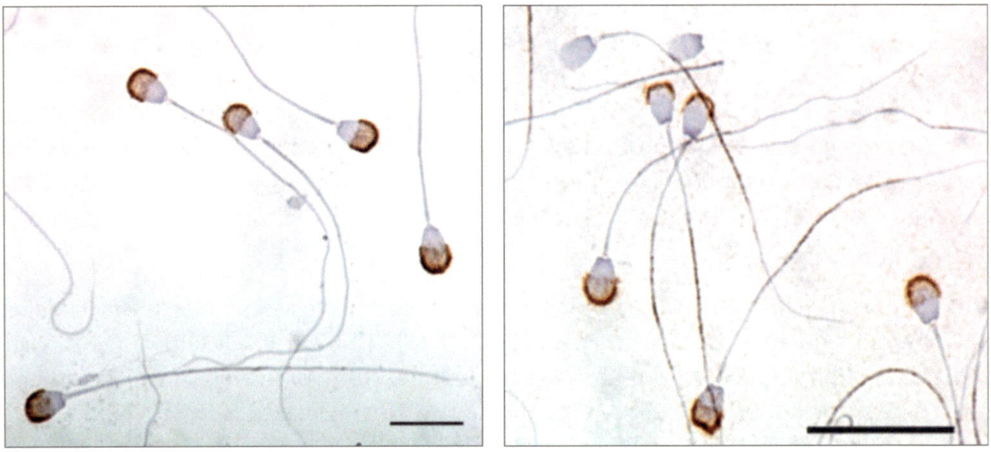

Figure 4. Canine sperm immunoreaction against HSP70 (Scale bar = 10 μm). In freshly ejaculated sperm (on the left), labelling for HSP70 is found over the acrosome region while the sperm tail is negative for this molecule. After freezing (on the right), a reduction of the intensity of immunostaining over the acrosome was found, with some negative sperm. In parallel, dislocation of the HSP immunoreactions to the sperm tail was observed.

3.3. Assessment of surface membrane integrity

Integrity of the sperm membrane is essential to sperm survival in the female genital tract and to fertilization [32]. Until placed in the female reproductive tract, spermatozoa are maintained in a hyperosmotic medium. Thereafter, it is passed into an iso-osmotic medium and contacts not only with the genital fluid, but also with the epithelia of the uterus and the uterine tubes, where it is stored. Further, molecules present on the sperm surface are of utmost significance for the spermatozoa interaction with the female local immune system, binding with the uterine tube epithelium, to cross the oocyte vestments (*cumulus* cells and *zona pellucida*) and to fertilize the oocyte. The molecular and hormonal local environment possess an important regulatory role on what concerns the sperm functions. However, to fulfil its role the sperm needs to acknowledge those influences and to react accordingly. Cell membrane damages are one of the major side effects of cryopreservation and are irreversible [33]. It is due to changes in the membrane structure and lateral phase separation of the membrane components leading to focal aggregation of proteins, disarrangement of the membrane lipids and increased permeability to solutes [11,33].

When introduced in a hypo- or hypertonic environment, cells tend to adjust and reach osmotic equilibrium by allowing water and solutes to change across the cell membrane. Spermatozoa, among other cells, have the ability to maintain their volume after osmotic shock [1,34]. It has for long been proved that, for domestic species, cell volume control shows a close positive correlation with fertility [1]. In the ejaculate, there is usually sperm with different aptitudes and with differences in the ability to respond to osmotic stressors. This is often related with membrane deficiencies in ion channels or signalling pathways that control cell volume. The ability to adapt to osmotic changes can be tested by the hypoosmotic test (HOST), an indirect method to assess the membrane integrity, where sperm is incubated in hypoosmotic solutions between 1-60 minutes at 37ºC. Spermatozoa with intact plasmalemma become swollen and present coiled tails when incubated in a sucrose solution (ranging from 75 to 150 mOsm, according to the species) (Figure 5). After longer exposures, they recover the initial volume [34]. Although currently used for *in vitro* semen assessment, this evaluation is subjective and not quantitatively rigorous. It is also possible that a number of sperm cells may die if prolonged incubation periods are used, biasing the results. However, it becomes more precise if performed with the aid of an electronic cell counter. In this approach, known as the volume regulatory test, after the osmotic challenge, sperm passes through a capillary pore and cell volume is determined upon changes in the electric resistance to passage. The results are expressed as cell frequency distribution for the iso- and the hypoosmotic moments of the test and the amount of displacement of the distribution curve, which reflects the adaptability of the sampled cells [1].

Different combinations of fluorescent membrane-impermeable dyes may also be used to assess the sperm membrane integrity. Most commonly used ones, also show some degree of affinity for DNA, as for Hoechst 33258, propidium iodide (PI) or ethidium homodimer 1 [11]. Alternatively acylated membrane dyes are also used. These dyes can cross the intact cell membrane and be held in the viable spermatozoa. When the plasma membrane is damaged, the probe leak out of the cell. More recently, fluorescein diacetate (CFDA), carboxyl(methil)-derivates, such as carboxyl-SNARF and SYBR-14 have been used for this purpose (for more detail, see [11]). This sort of probes can be combined and used with flow cytometry. The combination of different patterns allows estimating different degrees of sperm viability [13]. When combined with PI, green fluorochromes such as CFDA (Carboxyfluorescein diacetate) or SYBER-14 are replaced in the dead spermatozoa by the red fluorescence, which is not found in the membrane intact sperm. Carboxyl-SNARF, a pH-indicator, stains the live spermatozoa in orange, whilst Hoechst 33258 stains the dead spermatozoa in bright-blue [11].

Sperm membrane integrity can also be assessed by the use of merocyanine 540 (MC540), a hydrophylic probe with highly disorganized lipids that shows a high affinity pattern for instable membranes. This probe allows to monitor the changes in the cell membrane lipid architecture. Two sperm populations may be found under a fluorescent microscope: sperm with intact membranes devoid of fluorescence and sperm with disordered cell membranes that emit fluorescence [7,35]. This probe further labels sperm round, apoptotic bodies, which are more frequently found in men with decreased sperm quality [14]. Whether these structures are indicators of pathological or excessive apoptosis in the male genital tract or simply cell remnants of similar density to sperm heads is still to prove.

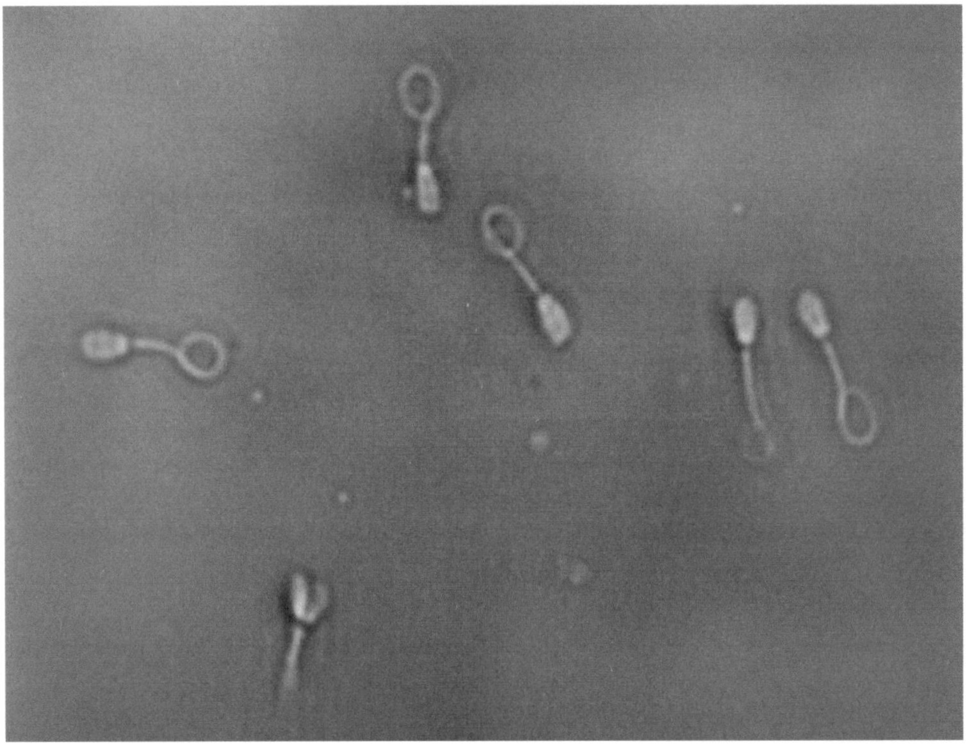

Figure 5. Canine spermatozoa in a HOST test (magnification 100x).

Besides the modifications on lipid arrangement in sperm plasma membrane, loss of membrane integrity also induces disorganization of the membrane proteins. In fact, in defective sperm or after cold-shock, the clustering of the membrane proteins is frequently observed. At fertilization, such modifications can interfere with the exposition of molecular epitopes and compromise receptor-ligand interactions between sperm and the oviductal cells or the oocyte [15,36]. A more conservative approach to test these changes includes the functional *in vitro* gamete interaction tests, such as the oocyte penetration test or the hemi-zona assay (for a quick review see [11]). The *zona pellucida* binding assay tests the ability of spermatozoa to interact with the *zona pellucida* of the oocytes. It is an assay with much variability and it tends to be replaced for the hemi-zona assay, which has the advantage of allowing the comparison between 2 sperm samples (one being used as control) on a single ovum. The oocyte penetration test assesses the fertilizing ability of spermatozoa by evaluating the presence of fluorescent spermatozoa heads in the perivitelline space and in the ooplasm after several hours of sperm-oocyte co-incubation [37].

Further, ICC, Western blotting, Chromatography and ELISA (Enzyme-linked immunosorbent assay) techniques can be used to detect the immunoexpression of particular membrane proteins (like integrins, adhesins or membrane-anchored proteases- ADAM) and to assess possible changes in immunoexpression in defective sperm following a challenging stimulus.

Recently, some studies have been presented, concerning the water channels function in spermatozoa and their functions in the cell volume regulation and sperm adaptation to environmental changes in osmotic pressure. Aquaporins (AQPs) are a family of proteins highly specialized in water permeability and involved in water transport across membranes. It has been demonstrated that AQP3 is an important water channel localized on the principal piece of the sperm tail, which acts like a key-fluid regulator for sperm osmoadaptation, protecting the cell membrane from swelling and mechanical stretching damages [38]. By using a fluorescence immunocytochemistry approach and flow cytometry, it was found that in AQP3 defective sperm exist an increased proportion of tail bending at cytoplasmic droplet under osmotic stressor conditions, which were associated to membrane rupture and exaggerated cell swelling during HOST, along with decreased sperm motility and reduced fertilization [38]. Additional AQP's have been localized on the sperm of different species. AQP7 and AQP8 may play a role in the glycerol metabolism and water transport respectively, with AQP7 showing some association with sperm progressive motility [39].

3.4. Assessment of the oxidative stress and apoptosis

Sperm metabolism in aerobic conditions originates oxidative molecules (reactive oxygen species or ROS - short-lived reactive chemical intermediates), which are highly reactive and oxidize lipids, proteins and glycides. Cells contribute to the maintenance of the oxidative homeostasis by controlling the amount of ROS, converting them into less injuring molecules [40,41]. Excessive ROS production damages the sperm membrane, reduces motility (by decreasing membrane potential), induces irreparable DNA damage and is closely associated with apoptosis [42,43]. Oxidation reaction in the membranes increases ROS, changes membrane fluidity and compromises its integrity, impairs ion-gradients and lipid-protein interaction and causes changes in proteins [44,45]. The seminal plasma possesses various natural antioxidants that protect spermatozoa against the oxidative stress which are removed when sperm is diluted or submitted to a process for preservation. Spermatozoa are particularly susceptible to lipid peroxidation, and one should be aware that semen manipulation and cryopreservation-thaw procedures accelerate the production of reactive oxygen species. Within the spermatozoa, mitochondria and the plasma membrane are the most sensitive structures to ROS [45].

Lipid peroxidation (LPO) releases membrane polyunsaturated fatty acids that are used as substrates for ROS and hydroxyl radical generation. The most frequent product of LPO is malonaldehyde (MDA) [44]. LPO can be indirectly assessed using a spectrophotometer by measuring thiobarbituric acid reactive (TBAR) substances; the method is based on the measurement of the complex formed by the reaction of MDA with TBA under a temperature stressor (incubation at 100ºC), which produce a pink-coloured chromogen and is readable at a wavelength of 532 nm. Also, the fluorescent probe BODIPY$^{581/591}$-C11 (4,4-difluoro-5-(4-phenyl-1,3-butadienyl)-4-bora-3a,4a-diaza-s-indacene-3-undecanoic acid) is frequently used in association with flow cytometry to assess LPO in the sperm. BODIPY is a fatty acids sensitive fluorescent probe that changes fluorescence from red to green in the presence of lipid peroxidation. Its association with a vital probe further allows to evaluate the fluorescence emission ratio in living cells [44,46].

Additional, currently used methods also include the glutathione peroxidase reaction (where the hydrogen peroxide oxidizes GSH (reduced glutathione) into GSSG (oxidized glutathione) in the presence of glutathione reductase and NADPH results from the consumption of NADPH in proportion to the peroxide content), by flow cytometry measurement of the fluorescent intensity of the compounds oxidized by ROS (such as the dichlorofluorescin diacetate- DCFH-DA- or the Hydroethidine- HE), using the gas-liquid chromatography separation of lipid peroxides, followed by its identification by mass spectrometry and by measuring cytotoxic aldehydes through high performance liquid chromatography (HPLC) [44,45].

ROS production can be directly monitored by a luminol or a lucigenin-based chemilluminescence assay [43,45]. This assay does not distinguish between intracellular and extracellular ROS, but it differentiates between the production of superoxide and hydrogen peroxide according to the probe used (lucigenin and luminol, respectively for superoxide and hydrogen peroxide). Measurement of chemilluminescence is proportional to ROS accumulation [45].

An important side effect of the oxidative stress is apoptosis [42]. The most important changes associated to sperm apoptosis are the externalization of the phosphatidylserine (PS), a molecule usually confined to the inner leaflet of the plasma membrane, the caspase system activation, the DNA fragmentation, the lost of mitochondrial integrity and the increase of cell membrane permeability [41]. To assess sperm apoptosis it is frequently used the Annexin V, a Ca^{2+}-dependent PS-binding protein that reacts to the PS, which is translocated to the outer leaflet of the plasma membrane in damaged sperm. Annexin V can be conjugated to fluorochromes such as FITC (Fluorescein isothiocyanate) in flow cytometry analysis. If a vital staining is used, such as the propidium iodide, the combination allows to distinguish between three sperm sub-populations: viable (Annexin-FITC-PI-negative), early apoptotic (Annexin-FITC-positive and PI-negative) and late apoptotic (Annexin-FITC-PI-positive) [7,41].

Caspases are molecules associated with the apoptotic pathway and can be classified as initiators or executors; caspase 7 and 9 are initiators, while active caspase 3 is an executor. The determination of the caspase enzymatic activity in sperm extracts, in comparison to the one of neutrophils, can also be used to assess apoptosis in sperm, which may be completed by the semiquantitative determination of active caspase 3 and caspase 7 content, by Western blotting. Caspase activity has been shown to be consistently higher in low motility sperm, in particular, the active caspase 3 [47].

Assessment of additional molecules known to be involved in the apoptosis mechanism, which might work as possible biological markers, can be performed by ICC, Western blotting or even in proteomic studies. Some molecules participating or regulating apoptotic processes in cells have been analysed in sperm and in semen, and its concentration was found to correlate with sperm quality. Among these molecules, TNF localization in pig and canine sperm has been performed [48,49]. The immunolabelling is limited to the sperm mid-piece in the mitochondrial region (Figure 6) and it has been demonstrated that a decrease in TNF immunoreaction is observed in spermatozoa incubated in a capacitating medium. When exposed to TNF, spermatozoa showed decreased motility, increased PS externalization and chromatin and DNA damage, changes that are usually associated with apoptosis [50].

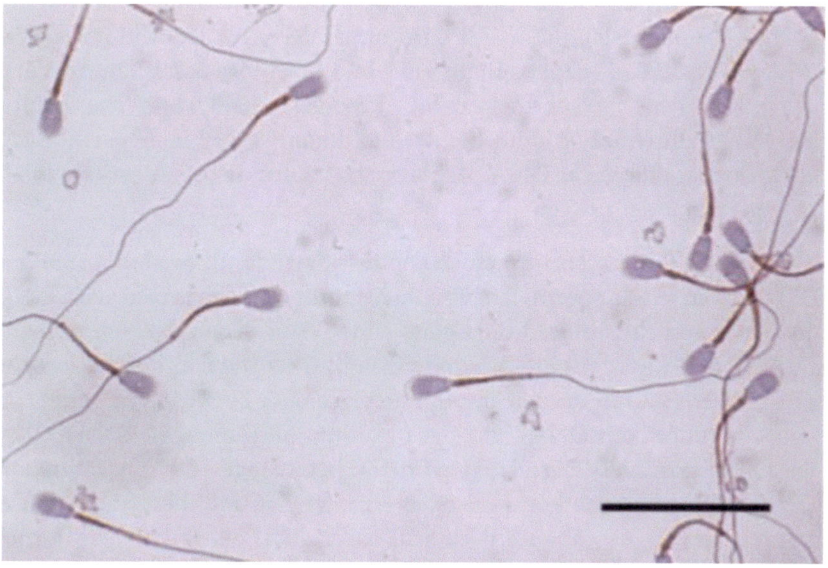

Figure 6. Sperm immunoreactions against TNF. In canine spermatozoa, strong immunolabelling for TNF was found in sperm mid–piece, in the mitochondrial region.

3.5. Assessment of DNA integrity

An association between infertility and the integrity of DNA content in sperm has been suggested. The integrity of male DNA is of utmost importance for embryo development and offspring production [13,41]. DNA damage is not usually perceived under classic or advanced semen assessment, but has been proposed to be at the origin of infertility in normospermic individuals. DNA damage (abnormal chromatin structure) may arise from different processes: deficient recombination or packaging during spermatogenesis, apoptosis and oxidative stress. DNA loss of integrity does not always impair fertilization, but compromises sustainable embryo development, predisposing to embryo losses and abortion [9,15]. DNA fragmentation may be associated with various pathological and environmental conditions [51,52], but also with endogenous mechanisms such as the oxidative stress and apoptosis.

Evaluation of sperm DNA integrity can be achieved by a variety of tests covering different aspects of the DNA damage. Unfortunately, most of the available techniques provide limited information regarding the nature of the DNA lesions evidenced, and do not allow to highlight the exact pathogenesis of disrupted sperm DNA [53,54].

Less expensive methods to assess the sperm chromatin structure uses chromatin structural probes or dyes, such as the acridine orange (measures the susceptibility to conformational changes), the aniline blue (that stains loosely condensed chromatin), chromomycin α (competing with protamine binding to DNA, it reveals protamination defects on sperm) and the toluidine blue (that stains phosphate residues of fragmented DNA). However, several factors modulate the DNA staining of chromatin, decreasing their specificity [52].

Nowadays, the most currently used tests of sperm DNA fragmentation are: the Comet assay (single cell gel electrophoresis), the TUNEL (terminal deoxynucleotidyl transferase-mediated dUTP (2′-deoxyuridine, 5′-triphosphate) nick end labelling) assay, the sperm chromatin structure assay (SCSA) and the sperm chromatin dispersion (SCD) test. The first three assays focus on the DNA fragmentation detection, while the last assay is a sperm nuclear matrix assay detecting possible deficient DNA repair or chromatin disorganization [43]. On table 1 we compare these methods.

The Comet assay is a fluorescence microscopic test that identifies single (SS) and double-stranded (DS) DNA in single sperm. In this assay, sperm cells are mixed with low-to-moderate melting agarose and then placed on a glass slide. The cells are lysed and then subjected to horizontal electrophoresis, the DNA being visualized with the aid of a fluorochrome dye. DNA damage is quantified by measuring the displacement between the genetic material of the comet nucleus (unbroken DNA) and the resulting tail (damaged DNA) [21,52,53]. The length of the tail is positively correlated with the percentage of DNA fragmentation. Although highly sensitive, this method is also labour intensive and the comet tail is of difficult standardization. Further, less apparent clinical association exists between the test results and clinical infertility [43], and clinical thresholds were yet to be established.

TUNEL assay is possibly the most common method used to assess sperm damage in sperm. It can be used as another ICC method, in both bright field and fluorescence microscopy, or associated with flow cytometry. In the TUNEL assay, terminal deoxynucleotidyl transferase (TdT) incorporates labelled nucleotides into 3′-OH at single- and double-strand DNA breaks, creating a signal of increasing intensity according to the number of DNA breaks. The fluorescence intensity of each analysed sperm is scored as a "positive" or "negative" on a microscope slide. When conjoined with a flow cytometer, precision of the method increases due to the increased number of cells analysed [43,53]. Proportion of TUNEL positive cells seems to be correlated with decreased pregnancy rates [13]. However, numerous variations for the test exist, which reduces its liability.

The sperm chromatin structure assay measures *in situ* DNA susceptibility to acid-induced DNA denaturation. It uses a flow cytometer and the acridine orange fluorescence, a traditional fluorescent dye that shows different colour when bonded to single- (red) or double-stranded (green) DNA [43]. The degree of red fluorescence in a sample (named DNA fragmentation index - DFI) has been associated to male infertility [13,43,53]. It is possible to score different spermatozoa populations by using SCSA: the sperm without fragmented DNA, the sperm with moderate DFI and the sperm with high DFI.

The sperm chromatin dispersion test (SCD) is a method based on the principle that sperm with fragmented DNA fail to produce a halo, which is characteristically observed in sperm with non-fragmented DNA, when mixed in aqueous, low melting agarose followed by acid denaturation and removal of nuclear proteins [21,54]. Despite not being necessary, this test can be visualised using a fluorescent dye (such as propidium iodide, DAPI or ethidium bromide) or simply be stained with Diff-Quick® reagent. Halosperm® is a commercial kit to assess DNA fragmentation in sperm from different species, before or after semen manipulation. Regarding this kit, sperm presenting a large- and medium-sized halo is considered to have no fragmentation, while spermatozoa having a small halo or without halo is classified as having DNA fragmentation (Figure 7) [55].

Assay	Parameter	Principle	Detection method
TUNEL	Addition of labeled dUTP nucleotides with deoxynucleotidyl transferase to SS and DS DNA breaks Template independent	Cells with labelled DNA (%)	Microscopy (bright or fluorescence) Flow cytometry
Comet	Fragmented DNA in sperm cells is detected by eletrophoresis Alkaline conditions denature DNA and reveals SS and DS DNA breaks Neutral conditions reveal mostly DS breaks	% cells with migration tails (fragmented DNA) and also the length of the tail (% DNA in the tail)	Fluorescence microscopy
SCSA	Mild acid treatment denaturates and lyses DNA with SS or DS breaks Acridine orange differentially emits fluorescence with DS DNA (Green) or SS DNA (Red)	DFI (%) = cells with red fluorescence divided by the total of cells (red+green).	Flow cytometry
SCD	Mild acid denaturation of DNA and lysis of protamines induce a decondensation halo around sperm head if DNA is intact, and no halo is observed if DNA is damaged	% Cells with small or no halo	Microscopy (bright or fluorescence)

Table 1. Comparison of available methods for assessment of DNA fragmentation is spermatozoa (Adapted from [56]). (SS- Single-stranded; DS- Double-stranded; DFI-DNA fragmentation index)

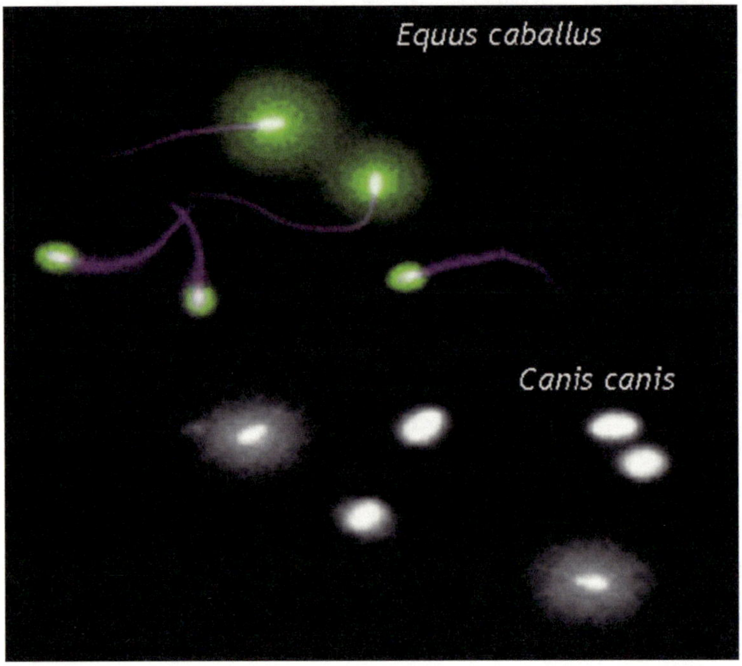

Figure 7. Image of the Halosperm® test for DNA fragmentation in horses and dogs. The existence of a large halo is indicative of DNA integrity (Adapted from [56]).

4. Concluding remarks

Conventional, currently methods used in sperm quality assessment are unsatisfactory to correctly predict sperm fertility potential and do not provide sufficient information for diagnosing and overcome some clinical infertility situations. The major advantages of biomarker approach over conventional semen analysis are the proficiency to accurately measure biomarker levels and to expose hidden sperm defects, which go undetected during current sperm morphology assessment. Newer, unconventional diagnostic tests of sperm function have the increased potential to deliver relevant information and to have an effective predictive role in male reproductive medicine. In the present work, several molecular markers have been presented for each of the sperm functions. Some are already used in human andrology, but are less used for the animals. Its use allows an increased efficiency in the identification of infertile individuals or to predict the sperm behaviour to manipulation, hence predicting the degree of damage to be expected for a given sperm sample. The development of test based on predicted sperm functions such as capacitation and in particular sperm–oocyte interaction will present increasing impact on the field of extenders research, as well as of semen banks implementation for both domestic and wild species. It is of utmost interest the characterization of a particular biomarker patterns/levels in fertile and infertile samples, with the subsequent ability to identify males with superior tolerance to semen cryopreservation. Nevertheless, putative molecular markers that may be used for sperm quality assessment were not exhausted in this review. Further efforts must be focused on understanding how these biomarkers correlate with transient impairments of male infertility caused by heat stress, malnutrition, diseases or trauma. Finally, the adjunctive evaluation of spermatozoa functions is particular important when considering sperm storage.

Acknowledgments

This work was supported by the project from CECAV/UTAD with the reference PEst-OE/AGR/UI0772/2011, by the Portuguese Science and Technology Foundation.

Author details

Rita Payan-Carreira[1*], Paulo Borges[1,2], Fernando Mir[2] and Alain Fontbonne[2]

*Address all correspondence to: rtpayan@gmail.com

1 CECAV [Veterinary and Animal Research Centre] – University of Trás-os-Montes and Alto Douro, Vila Real, Portugal

2 CERCA (Centre d'Études en Reproduction des Carnivores), Animal Reproduction, National Veterinary School of Alfort, Paris-East University, France

References

[1] Petrunkina AM, Waberski D, Günzel-Apel AR, Töpfer-Petersen E. Determinants of sperm quality and fertility in domestic species. Reproduction. 2007, 134: 3-17

[2] Sutovsky P, Lovercamp K. Molecular markers of sperm quality. Soc Reprod Fertil Suppl. 2010, 67: 247-56.

[3] Dyck MK, Foxcroft GR, Novak S, Ruiz-Sanchez A, Patterson J, Dixon WT. Biological markers of boar fertility. Reprod Domest Anim. 2011, 46 (Suppl 2): 55-8.

[4] Mortimer ST. A critical review of the physiological importance and analysis of sperm movement in mammals. Hum Reprod Update. 1997, 3: 403-39.

[5] Payan-Carreira R, Miranda S and Nizanski W. Artificial Insemination in Dogs. In: Artificial Insemination in Farm Animals. Milad Manafi (Ed.), 2011. ISBN: 978-953-307-312-5, InTech, Available from: http://www.intechopen.com/books/artificial-insemination-in-farm-animals/artificial-insemination-in-dogs

[6] Lefièvre L, Bedu-Addo K, Conner SJ, Machado-Oliveira GS, Chen Y, Kirkman-Brown JC, Afnan MA, Publicover SJ, Ford WC, Barratt CL. Counting sperm does not add up any more: time for a new equation? Reproduction. 2007, 133:675-84.

[7] Ramalho-Santos J, Amaral A, Sousa AP, Rodrigues AS, Martins L, Baptista M, Mota PC, Tavares R, Amaral S, Gamboa S. Probing the structure and function of mammalian sperm using optical and fluorescence microscopy. In: Modern Research and Educational Topics in Microscopy. A Mendez-Villas and J Diaz (Eds.), 2007. Badajoz, Spain: FORMATEX. Pp: 394-402.

[8] Heriberto Rodriguez-Martinez. Cryopreservation of Porcine Gametes, Embryos and Genital Tissues: State of the Art. In: Current Frontiers in Cryobiology, Igor I. Katkov (Ed.), 2012. ISBN: 978-953-51-0191-8, InTech, Available from: http://www.intechopen.com/books/current-frontiers-in-cryobiology/cryopreservation-of-pig-spermatozoa-oocytes-and-embryos-state-of-the-art.

[9] Watson PF. The causes of reduced fertility with cryopreserved semen. Anim Reprod Sci. 2000, 60-61:481-92.

[10] Pesch S, Hoffmann B. J. Reproduktionsmed. Cryopreservation of Spermatozoa in Veterinary Medicine. Endokrinol. 2007, 4: 101-105

[11] Partyka A, Niżański W and Ochota M. Methods of Assessment of Cryopreserved Semen, Current Frontiers in Cryobiology, Igor I. Katkov (Ed.), 2012. ISBN: 978-953-51-0191-8, InTech, Available from: http://www.intechopen.com/books/current-frontiers-in-cryobiology/methods-of-assessment-of-cryopreserved-semen

[12] Kim SH, Yu DH, Kim YJ. Apoptosis-like change, ROS, and DNA status in cryopreserved canine sperm recovered by glass wool filtration and Percoll gradient centrifugation techniques. Anim Reprod Sci. 2010, 119:106-14.

[13] Silva PF, Gadella BM. Detection of damage in mammalian sperm cells. Theriogenology. 2006, 65:958-78.

[14] Muratori M, Luconi M, Marchiani S, Forti G, Baldi E. Molecular markers of human sperm functions. Int J Androl. 2009, 32:25-45.

[15] Samplaski MK, Agarwal A, Sharma R, Sabanegh E. New generation of diagnostic tests for infertility: review of specialized semen tests. Int J Urol. 2010, 17:839-47.

[16] Rodriguez-Martinez H. Role of the oviduct in sperm capacitation. Theriogenology. 2007, 68 (Suppl 1):S138-46.

[17] Costello S, Michelangeli F, Nash K, Lefievre L, Morris J, Machado-Oliveira G, Barratt C, Kirkman-Brown J, Publicover S. Ca2+-stores in sperm: their identities and functions. Reproduction. 2009, 138:425-37.

[18] Graham JK.Assessment of sperm quality: a flow cytometric approach. Anim Reprod Sci. 2001, 68:239-47.

[19] Strünker T, Goodwin N, Brenker C, Kashikar ND, Weyand I, Seifert R, Kaupp UB. The CatSper channel mediates progesterone-induced Ca2+ influx in human sperm. Nature. 2011, 471:382-6.

[20] Makkar G, Ng EH, Yeung WS, Ho PC. The significance of the ionophore-challenged acrosome reaction in the prediction of successful outcome of controlled ovarian stimulation and intrauterine insemination. Hum Reprod. 2003, 18:534-9.

[21] Memili E, Dogan S, Rodriguez-Osorio E, Wang X, de Oliveira RV, Mason MC, Govindaraju A, Grant KE, Belser LE, Crate E, Moura A, Kaya A. Makings of the Best Spermatozoa: Molecular Determinants of High Fertility. In: Male Infertility, Anu Bashamboo and Kenneth David McElreavey (Ed.), 2012. ISBN: 978-953-51-0562-6, InTech,. Available from: http://www.intechopen.com/books/male-infertility/makings-of-the-best-spermatozoa-molecular-determinants-of-high-fertility

[22] Oliva R, de Mateo S, Estanyol JM. Sperm cell proteomics. Proteomics. 2009, 9:1004-17.

[23] Brewis IA, Gadella BM. Sperm surface proteomics: from protein lists to biological function. Mol Hum Reprod. 2010, 16:68-79.

[24] Berlinguer F, Madeddu M, Pasciu V, Succu S, Spezzigu A, Satta V, Mereu P, Leoni GG, Naitana S. Semen molecular and cellular features: these parameters can reliably predict subsequent ART outcome in a goat model. Reprod Biol Endocrinol. 2009, 7:125

[25] Sousa AP, Amaral A, Baptista M, Tavares R, Caballero Campo P, Caballero Peregrín P, Freitas A, Paiva A, Almeida-Santos T, Ramalho-Santos J. Not all sperm are equal: functional mitochondria characterize a subpopulation of human sperm with better fertilization potential. PLoS One. 2011 6:e18112. doi:10.1371/journal.pone.0018112.

[26] Liu DY, Clarke GN, Baker HW. Hyper-osmotic condition enhances protein tyrosine phosphorylation and zona pellucida binding capacity of human sperm. Hum Reprod. 2006, 21: 745-752.

[27] Cole JA, Meyers SA. Osmotic stress stimulates phosphorylation and cellular expression of heat shock proteins in rhesus macaque sperm. J Androl. 2011, 32:402-10.

[28] Ecroyd H, Jones RC, Aitken RJ. Tyrosine phosphorylation of HSP-90 during mammalian sperm capacitation. Biol Reprod. 2003, 69:1801-7.

[29] Spinaci M, Vallorani C, Bucci D, Bernardini C, Tamanini C, Seren E, Galeati G. Effect of liquid storage on sorted boar spermatozoa. Theriogenology. 2010, 74:741-8.

[30] Borges P, Mir F, Fontbonne A, Carreira R, "Study of HSP70 expression in dog semen submitted to cold-thermal treatment". Book of Abstracts of the European Veterinary Conference - Voorjaarsdagen, 5 to 7 April 2012, Amsterdam, The Netherlands: 249-250

[31] Borges P, Mir F, Fontbonne A, Carreira R. [HSP70 Redistribution in canine spermatozoa after chilling and freezing] (In portuguese) Abstract book of the V Congresso da

Sociedade Portuguesa de Ciências Veterinárias, 13-15 October 2011, Fonte Boa, Portugal: 164.

[32] Holt, W.V. Fundamental aspects of sperm cryobiology: the importance of species and individual differences. Theriogenology 2000, 53: 47-58.

[33] Meyers SA. Spermatozoal response to osmotic stress. Anim Reprod Sci. 2005, 89:57-64.

[34] England GC, Plummer JM. Hypo-osmotic swelling of dog spermatozoa. J Reprod Fertil. 1993, Suppl. 47:261-70.

[35] Hallap T, Nagy S, Jaakma U, Johannisson A, Rodriguez-Martinez H. Usefulness of a triple fluorochrome combination Merocyanine 540/Yo-Pro 1/Hoechst 33342 in assessing membrane stability of viable frozen-thawed spermatozoa from Estonian Holstein AI bulls. Theriogenology. 2006, 65:1122-36.

[36] Rajeev SK, Reddy KV. Sperm membrane protein profiles of fertile and infertile men: identification and characterization of fertility-associated sperm antigen. Hum Reprod. 2004, 19:234-42.

[37] Hewitt, D.A., England, G.C.W. The canine oocyte penetration assay; its use as an indicator of dog spermatozoa performance in vitro. Anim Reprod Sci. 1997, 50:123-139.

[38] Chen Q, Peng H, Lei L, Zhang Y, Kuang H, Cao Y, Shi QX, Ma T, Duan E. Aquaporin3 is a sperm water channel essential for postcopulatory sperm osmoadaptation and migration.Cell Res. 2011, 21:922-33.

[39] Yeung CH, Callies C, Tüttelmann F, Kliesch S, Cooper TG. Aquaporins in the human testis and spermatozoa - identification, involvement in sperm volume regulation and clinical relevance. Int J Androl. 2010, 33:629-41.

[40] Garrido N, Meseguer M, Simon C, Pellicer A, Remohi J. Pro-oxidative and anti-oxidative imbalance in human semen and its relation with male fertility. Asian J Androl. 2004, 6:59-65.

[41] Agarwal A, Varghese AC, Sharma RK. Markers of oxidative stress and sperm chromatin integrity. Methods Mol Biol. 2009, 590:377–402

[42] Kim, S-H., Yu D-H. & KimY-J. Effects of cryopreservation on phosphatidylserine translocation, intracellular hydrogen peroxide, and DNA integrity in canine sperm. Theriogenology. 2010, 73:282–292.

[43] Natali A, Turek PJ. An assessment of new sperm tests for male infertility. Urology. 2011, 77:1027-34.

[44] Sanocka D, Kurpisz M. Reactive oxygen species and sperm cells. Reprod Biol Endocrinol. 2004, 2:12.

[45] Agarwal A, Makker K, Sharma R. Clinical relevance of oxidative stress in male factor infertility: an update. Am J Reprod Immunol. 2008, 59:2-11.

[46] Gallardo Bolaños JM, Morán AM, Balao da Silva CM, Morillo Rodríguez A, Plaza Dávila M, Aparicio IM, Tapia JA, Ortega Ferrusola C, Peña FJ. Autophagy and Apoptosis Have a Role in the Survival or Death of Stallion Spermatozoa during Conservation in Refrigeration. 2012 PLoS ONE 7(1):e30688. doi:10.1371/journal.pone.0030688.

[47] Taylor SL, Weng SL, Fox P, Duran EH, Morshedi MS, Oehninger S, Beebe SJ. Somatic cell apoptosis markers and pathways in human ejaculated sperm: potential utility as indicators of sperm quality. Mol Hum Reprod. 2004, 10:825-34.

[48] Payan-Carreira R, Santana I, Pires MA, Holst BS, Rodriguez-Martinez H. Localization of tumor necrosis factor in the canine testis, epididymis and spermatozoa. Theriogenology. 2012, 77:1540-8

[49] Payan-Carreira R, Siqueira A, Gonzalez Herrero R "TNF immunolocalization in boar spermatozoa". Reprod Dom Anim. 2011, 46 (Suppl. 3): 72

[50] Perdichizzi A, Nicoletti F, La Vignera S, Barone N, D'Agata R, Vicari E, Calogero AE. Effects of tumour necrosis factor-alpha on human sperm motility and apoptosis. J Clin Immunol. 2007, 27:152-62.

[51] Zini A, Libman J. Sperm DNA damage: clinical significance in the era of assisted reproduction. CMAJ. 2006, 175:495-500.

[52] Evenson D, Wixon R. Meta-analysis of sperm DNA fragmentation using the sperm chromatin structure assay. Reprod Biomed Online. 2006, 12:466-72.

[53] Bungum M. Sperm DNA integrity assessment: a new tool in diagnosis and treatment of fertility. Obstet Gynecol Int. 2012, 2012:531042.

[54] Agarwal A, Said TM Sperm chromatin assessment. In Textbook of ART (2nd Ed.) DK Gardner, A Weissman, CM Howles, A Shoham (Edt), 2004. PLC (Taylor and Francis Group) London, UK: pp 93–106.

[55] Yılmaz S, Zergeroğlu AD, Yılmaz E, Sofuoglu K, Delikara N, Kutlu P. Effects of Sperm DNA Fragmentation on Semen Parameters and ICSI Outcome Determined by an Improved SCD Test, Halosperm. International Jourtal of Fertility and Sterility 2010 4(2): 73-78.

[56] Halotech DNA SL - www.halotechdna.com/products/halosperm [Assessed in 14-07-2012]

Chapter 7

The Potential for Infectious Disease Contamination During the Artificial Insemination Procedure in Swine

Emílio César Martins Pereira, Abelardo Silva Júnior,
Eduardo Paulino da Costa and
Carlos Eduardo Real Pereira

Additional information is available at the end of the chapter

http://dx.doi.org/10.5772/52337

1. Introduction

The productivity of the swine confinement has been steadily increasing in the last years. According to data from [1], the largest producer of pork is China, which is responsible for producing 49.5 million tons and is followed by the European Union, United States and Brazil (22.5; 10.2 and 3.2 million tons, respectively). The increased productivity of the swine meat is mainly related to the use of technology in the genetics, nutrition, health and reproduction areas. The adoption of the artificial insemination (AI) in pigs from the 70-ies has been significantly contributing to the development of swine production [2].

AI has contributed to the increase of animal production, since it accelerates the dissemination of desirable characteristics from genetically superior animals. Worldwide, it is believed that 90% animals raised commercially are inseminated and this number is expected to further increase [3]. Thus, this biotechnology has been investigated in order to ensure best production indexes. These are supported by high rates of pregnancy and commercialization of the semen doses has been found, such as the creation of AI centrals in Denmark, Canada and Netherlands, which totalized exports to 35 countries in 2010.

The health issue and the difficulty of cryopreservation of the doses are considered as the main barriers to commercialization of doses from boar semen. Numerous studies have been carried out in order to develop efficient cryopreservation protocols, since this is the main method to ensure the maintenance of viable doses for a long period, as allowing for their transportation to long distances. Initially, the objective concerning AI was to obtain a better control over the sanitary conditions. However, it was noted that the considerable development of this biotechnology was not accompanied by scientific knowledge related to the transmission of diseases. On one hand, the use of the artificial insemination has the great advantage in optimizing the use of the boar, whereas reducing the number of animals in the farm and consequently the costs of the management, medicines and animal acquisitions, the AI may function as a means diffusing pathogens, since there is no ideal sanitary control during the collection and manipulation of the semen. In this case, the AI using contaminated semen just maximizing spread of certain virus and bacteria since a single boar ejaculate can be used for insemination of various sows.

In this context, a considerable concern is assumed in relation to hygienic procedures in the semen manipulation process, especially in relation to semen destined for international market [3]. This fact is justified by the evidence of the possibility for transmission of some diseases via semen of swine. Among the possible agents that can transmit diseases are Aujeszky's disease virus, *classical swine fever virus* (CSFV), *african swine fever virus, porcine circovirus 2* (PCV2), *porcine reproductive and respiratory syndrome virus* (PRRSV), *porcine parvovirus* (PPV), *Chlamydia* sp., *Leptospira* sp, *Mycobacterium tuberculosis, Mycobacterium paratuberculosis* and *Brucella abortus* [4].

The effect from contamination of the boar´s semen may represent a considerable economical loss to the producer. This occurs because the presence of the bacterial or viral agents in the semen leads to the loss of fertility and reduction of the semen quality in male, and embryonic/fetal death, endometritis and systemic infection in the inseminated females, thereby contributing to reduction in the size of the litters.

Although the routine addition of antibiotics (ATB) in the seminal diluents may even eliminate a high number of contaminant bacteria, most viral agents still remain alive. Therefore, a concern has been assumed in relation to those pathogenic agents. Despite the availability of studies concerning to antivirus, these ones are still not used commercially due to ineffectiveness of the action, especially related to high toxicity to sperm cells. Thus, the main control criteria AI are limited to veterinary communication, inspection by health agencies and control strategies such as vaccination, isolation and monitoring of animals [5]. Moreover, efficient routine tests for identification of contaminants in the semen samples still remain as a reality that is very far from the existent commercial farms.

Thus, this chapter aims to clarify some points referring to the potential for contamination by infectious agents during AI procedure in pigs, as well as to identify the main agents likely to be transmitted by this biotech, which can contribute to reduced fertility of the animals, besides the possible control measures that should be performed in order to reduce the dissemination and effect of those pathogens on animals.

2. Main risky points during Artificial Insemination (AI)

IA is a commercially widespread technique worldwide. Therefore, the procedure for collection and manipulation of the semen besides the AI itself must be carefully accomplished in order to ensure that AI will not represent a risky factor for transmission of infectious diseases. Although there are wide variety of diseases that could contaminate the semen and consequently the inseminated female, the significance of a particular disease will vary according to epidemiological parameters and geographical localization of the farm. Even the risk for disease transmission is not the same in different countries of the world. Hence, the concept of pathogen-free centrals has become a common cause, since it is possible to obtain the pathogen-free semen either in countries that are free and in those that are not free from certain disease, according to definition by World Organization for Animal Health (OIE).

Guérin and Pozzi, (2005) [6] suggested that diseases able to cause negative impact on AI can be evaluated according to health risk as follows: a) Diseases that were eradicated within a country or continent, such as the Classical Swine Fever in Brazil; b) diseases to which there is already an integrated program for control in AI, such as the CSFV or Aujeszky's disease, which implies a negative state of the donor boars; c) diseases that are considered as likely to be transmitted by AI, such as diseases associated with PCV2, PPV and transmissible gastroenteritis, which are neither controlled nor associated with prophylactic measures routinely adopted.

The seminal contamination may be classified as extrinsic or intrinsic. The first case occurs when contamination occurs through an external source, such as feces or contaminated materials used during semen collection or processing. The intrinsic contamination occurs due to viral infection that can be systemic or local, as occasioning viral elimination through testicles, accessory or preputial glands [6]. Thus, it can be indicated that the main risk points for contamination of the semen can occur at the semen collection stages, in semen manipulation, or in artificial insemination procedure according to sanitary conditions of the farm.

Before the semen collection procedure, all utensils to be used and specially the material in contact with the semen must be sterilized according to routine hygienic procedures and equipments available at each AI station. The use of dry heat (ovens), moist heat (autoclave) and radiation (ultraviolet) are most suitable for sterilization. These materials include the collecting funnel and the collecting glass where the semen will be stored until the moment of dilution. Because accidents may occur during the collection procedure, it is advisable to build up a stock of sterile materials ready to be used in the case of contamination during the procedure.

The animal' prepuce is usually contaminated by a wide variety of infectious agents, as reported by some authors [7,8,11]. Thus, the occurrence of agents such as *Corynebacterium suis, Arcobacter spp.* and the Aujeszky's disease virus (ADV) in the ejaculate of the infected animals becomes a real possibility to be considered. Therefore, the examination of the semen-donor animals prior to collection of the semen is essential in order to ensure the sanitary quality of the semen. However, this previous evaluation may be not completely effective. This is due to the fact that certain viral agents, such as ADV which causes the Aujeszky's disease, have the peculiar ability to establish latency in the reproductive organs, therefore causing contamination of the semen although the animals remain serologically negative for those diseases [9]. Other viral agents such as PCV2 and PRRSV have a determinated sero-conversion period over which the agent will be eliminated through semen. Even when the animal is serum-negative for the infection [10], this elimination may still occur under continuous or intermittent way during the months after infection [12]. Another measure that can be taken in order to reduce contamination is the elimination of the first ejaculatory jets, that are characterized by high microbial contamination, therefore obtaining a better quality of the semen. The environmental contamination is also a factor to be considered during the collection procedure. Thus, the sanitary procedure of either male' preputial region and the dummy sow used for collection are routine procedures to avoid an eventual contamination of the semen outside the animal' body.

When processing the semen, certain hygienic precautions should be taken during its dilution and straw filling in order to prevent contamination. Regardless of the viral source, the storage and manipulation conditions are fundamental to predict the potential risk for contamination of the semen. It is known that the fresh semen is favorable to preservation and dissemination of the virus between species [6]. Therefore, the places where they will be in contact with the semen should be thoroughly sterilized to prevent contamination. There is a false impression that the antibiotics present in diluents can prevent bacterial contamination, but this detail should be cautiously considered, since the antibiotic doses contained in the seminal diluents might contain only the bacterial proliferation and are ineffective against some specific strains and virus [13].

Another factor to be considered is the insemination procedure itself. During AI, the main contaminative source is the feces, which is contaminated mainly by *Porcine sapelovirus*. Therefore, the care related to washing of the perianal region should be reinforced in order to avoid contamination. Other agents which may be found in the feces such as *Escherichia coli*, *Salmonella sp.*, *Rotavirus A*, Porcine Adenovirus, when introduced into uterus through insemination pipette, may cause the infection of the uterus and consequently leads to reduction of fertility and litter size.

Concerning to the intrinsic contamination forms, many local and systemic diseases may move towards the reproductive tract and are transmitted via semen. Those diseases can be divided into viral and bacterial diseases. In relation to viral diseases, some have more potential risk for transmission, as presented in Table 1.

Most diseases that affect the reproductive tract and are caused by viral agents rather provoke classical clinical signs that serve as parameters for isolation of the animals besides avoiding the animal reproduction. However, some diseases may be transmitted via breeding, even when the animal shows no clinical signs becoming an even greater problem, since it is not possible to identify the infected animal [14]. It is believed that the period over which there is greater release of viral load is when the animal shows the clinical stage of the disease [15].

In cases of the appearance of clinical signs, generally the males are not used for reproduction. Furthermore, the males usually refuse to make the natural mating during those situations. In addition, there is the guarantee of the reduced risk for transmission the disease, unlike when there is no apparent infection. Finally, the insemination of the sows infected with a semen does not necessarily result into contamination of the female and the onset of the clinical disease in the same one. Thus, the complexity of the conditions required for establishment of this process were experimentally proved.

Agent	Virus Isolation in Semen	Potential risk for contamination
Porcine adenovirus	+	Low
Aujeszky diseasevirus	+	+
African swine fever virus	+	+
Blue eye disease virus	+	+
CSFV	+	+
Porcine sapelovirus	+	+
FMDV	+	Low
Influenza virus	+	Low
PCV2	+	+
PPV	+	+
PRRSV	+	+
Reovirus	+	Low
SPV	ND	+
SVD	+	+
TGEV	+	Very Low

Table 1. Presence of the viral agents in semen of pigs and the risk for their transmission through AI (Adapted from [14] and [6]. ND: No data; CSFV:*classical swine fever virus*; FMD: *foot and mouth disease virus*; PCV2: *porcine circovirus 2*; PPV: *porcine parvovirus*; PRRSV: *porcine reproductive and respiratory syndrome virus*; SPV: swine papilloma virus; SVD: swine vesicular disease virus; TGEV: transmissible gastroenteritis virus.

Depending on pathogen, other less important forms of the seminal contamination should be considered. Among them, it can mentioned the transmission through aerosols, urine, fomites, people, vectorial insects, birds and wild mammals [5].

Finally, for complete determination of the level for the disease transmission risk in a farm, the hygienic and sanitary standards adopted in this farm should not be disregarded. In practice, it is observed that farms which do not provide effective vaccination programs and present failures in sanitary practices are more subject to contamination of the animals. The animals under these environmental conditions face a constant challenge.

3. Major contaminants of semen during AI procedure

With the high spread of the AI technique, semen has become an important vehicle for dissemination of pathogenic agents, either by previous infection of the male' reproductive tract or by contamination of the ejaculate through inadequate hygiene of the person collecting, direct contact with animal's feces or even the use of contaminated diluents. Several agents such as viral or bacterial, may be present in semen or may contaminate it after ejaculation.

3.1. Bacterial contaminants

Naturally, the pig' fresh semen contains approximately 10^4 to 10^5 bacteria/ml [16]. Although those bacteria are not pathogenic, they present spermicidal effect, especially when they are present at high concentrations [17]. To aggravate the situation, the majority of the bacteria which may be present in semen have innate or acquired resistance to antimicrobial agents added to diluters of the semen [18]. Many antimicrobial agents may still have their optimum action impaired by environmental conditions, such as the temperature [19]. Therefore, even with addition of antibiotics, the bacterial transmission through AI is a situation that may occur.

Common bacteria which are associated with infections of the sows´ genital tract and are possibly transmitted via semen are presented below.

3.1.1. Leptospira spp.

Spirochetes of the Leptospira genus are the agents causing leptospirosis, a disease mainly characterized by reproductive disorders. In serological study conducted in Brazil, Favero et al. [20] (2002) observed that the most prevalent serovars associated with Leptospirosis are: pomona, icterohaemorrhagiae, copenhageni and tarassovi. The disease has worldwide distribution and leads to infertility of the animals [21].

The main route for elimination of the Leptospires is through urinary system [22]. However, they may be present in the infected animals´ semen, as causing the infection of the female and can lead to reproductive complications during the bacteremia phase, inclusive abortion [23]. The bacteria can persist in the kidneys and reproductive organs of both males and females, therefore facilitating the dissemination of the disease in herd, requiring an early diagnosis of the disease.

To fill out this need, the tests for antibody detection by serology are effective. However, for serotyping the Leptospires is necessary to consider other diagnostic techniques. Attention should be given to the vaccinated seropositivos animals, since the antibodies are likely due to vaccinal reaction. For detection of the agent, molecular tests can be performed by PCR and immunoassay such as the direct immunofluorescence [24, 25].

In the case of a positive diagnosis, even with few affected animals, the control must be taken by adopting the following criteria: management, fight against rodents, vaccination and drug treatment in order to prevent the dissemination of the disease in the herd. Considering that Leptospira are sensitive to a wide variety of antimicrobial agents, the treatment associated with vaccination and sanitary measures provides an effective control of the disease [26].

3.1.2. *Mycobacterium sp.*

Bacteria of the Mycobacterium genus are agents causing tuberculosis, a disease characterized by provoking granulomatous lesions in various organs. In pig herds, *Mycobacterium avium* is the most prevalent species, but infections caused by *Mycobacterium tuberculosis* and *Mycobacterium bovis* can also occur [27]. Although pulmonary tuberculosis is the commonest form, the dissemination of the infection by several other organs can occur in a form so-called milliary tuberculosis [28].

When the disease appears under milliary form, the granulomatous lesions may be present in the reproductive organs with caseous necrosis with areas of calcification in the testis and epididymis, therefore the elimination of the microorganisms by semen will occur [29, 30].

Those lesions associated with confirmatory tests, by using special colorations to identify the alcohol-acid resistant bacilli are sufficient for definitive diagnosis of the disease. For characterization of the species, the PCR technique has been used since the isolation of the mycobacterium strains is considered as laborious procedure [31, 32].

The possible sources of infection can be determined by characterization of the agent. Thus, the complete and definitive diagnosis is very important to the control. Moreover, the issues concerning the farm hygiene are factors to be considered because the exposure to feces are the main factor for infection and dissemination of the disease [33].

3.1.3. *Brucella suis*

The etiologic agent of brucellosis in pigs is the *Brucella suis*. The disease is characterized by high morbidity and reproductive disorders such as abortion, endometritis and placentitis in females and orchitis, changes of accessory glands, libido loss and infertility in male [34]. Abortion has been observed at 17 days after female cover with males which are positive for B. suis in semen. Infertility in animals is mainly due to the involvement of testicular structures and lack of libido in the infected animals. The cases of contamination of the accessory glands are even more critical, since the animals remain fertile and can disseminate high loads of B. suis in semen during prolonged periods.

It is an extremely important disease for countries of the South America, Asia and Africa, where it is totally widespread. In the countries of North America and European Union, the prevalence is low or the disease has been eradicated [19]. The main route for elimination of brucellosis in farms is the genital arising from a positive male which eliminates the microorganism in the semen. Bacteria reach the reproductive organs after invasion of the lymph nodes followed by bacteremia [35]. In male, the infection may persist throughout life. Thus, it is necessary to eliminate the positive animals to prevent the dissemination of the disease.

In the case of positive farms, the control procedures should be performed. Among them, the sanitary break after the elimination of the positive animals and the monitoring of the reproducers' serological profile has proved to be effective for elimination of the agent of the herd. Although, nowadays, the sanitary conditions in commercial farms and the agility of the definitive diagnosis have evolved considerably, some pathogens have generated insignificant infection levels, such as the case of *B. suis*.

The definitive diagnosis is accomplished through isolation of the agent. Although very specific, it is complex and expensive, as requiring efficient and alternative methods. Serology can be used but must be associated with confirmatory tests such as rivanol, 2-mercaptoethanol and complement fixation. Another possibility is the molecular diagnosis by PCR [36].

3.1.4. Chlamydia sp.

Chlamydiosis is a disease with worldwide distribution that affects several species of mammals and especially birds. The main species causing disease is Chlamydia psittaci [37] and it is associated with pneumonia, conjunctivitis, enteritis, arthritis, pericarditis, orchitis and uterine infections, as being the last two related to cases of perinatal abortion and stillbirths [38].

The microorganism can enter through digestive, respiratory or venereal via and multiply in the epithelial cells that are carried by macrophages and disseminate by the chain of regional lymph nodes and remaining unapparent, but sometimes causes diseases in organs nearby routes for entrance of the agent. In genital infections, the semen may be contaminated and it is responsible for birth of the weak (which eliminate the bacteria during long period, therefore they are an important vehicle for horizontal transmission of infection [39].

For diagnostic purposes, several serological tests can be performed and the agent detection can be performed through the isolation and PCR. However, fecal sample has little diagnostic value because studies have demonstrated the presence of Chlamydia in healthy pigs [40].

Although the main dissemination sources to be the asymptomatic animals, the infected animals showing clinical signs of disease should be isolated and treated [41]. It is important to avoid the contact of pigs with birds and other species that are susceptible to Chlamydiosis.

3.2. Viral contaminants of semen

Recently, a high number of viral agents have been detected in the semen of pigs. Those agents are mainly associated with reduction of the animal's reproductive performance and fertility problems [6]. Usually, the infections by virus is source of major concern to the swine producer than bacterial infections. This fact is due to characteristics of the viral agents, which can be eliminated at high loads before the first signs of the illness or when the signs are mild or unapparent, as causing a significant epidemiological problem. However, it is believed the high virus load to be only removed via semen during viremia. During this period, the breeding male presents clinical signs, therefore it is generally removed. In any way, the control procedures are hindered because the animals can continue to eliminate the virus after disappearance of the signs. In addition, the efficacy of the available commercial antiviral products are not commercially proved and may exhibit a high toxicity level to the semen.

Some major viral agents, which may be present in the genital tract and eliminated through semen, are summarized in the sequence.

3.2.1. *Porcine reproductive and respiratory syndrome virus (PRRSV)*

The PRRS is a disease characterized by reproductive failures and respiratory diseases caused by PRRS virus. After infection, the virus elimination period can last up to three months [12] which enables the virus to disseminate regionally, nationally and internationally through transit of the infected animals.

During this period, the discharge can occur by several routes, as the semen being among the principal ones, what results into infection of the female and reproduction failures. In the body, the virus multiplies in macrophages and establishes the first viremia and can reach various organs and systems, as including the reproductive tract. In female, it crosses the placental barrier and results into miscarriages and birth of weak piglets, which will be disseminators of the virus in herd [42]. The virus can be eliminated in the semen even in absence of the viremia and in presence of the neutralizing antibodies [43].

The changes in the semen contaminated with PRRSV present individual characteristics, with substantial quality loss through reduced motility, increased percentage of abnormal acrosomes and increase of the spermatozoids with altered morphology [44] as those spermatic pathologies being an indication for infection with PRRSV.

Complementing the clinical signs and spermatic changes, the serological techniques are effective for definitive diagnosis. However, those techniques indicate exposure to the agent without the guarantee of the presence of infection and the vaccinated animals have higher levels of antibodies, what may lead to false-positive results [45]. The viral isolation, RT-PCR and immunohistochemistry techniques are employed for the diagnosis of PRRS in which the virus is detected [46-48].

To control the disease, the commercial vaccines are effective in reducing the viral load from the infected animals [49]. In countries where there are no reports of the disease, the monitoring programs of the entry of animals and semen should be well established and rigid.

3.2.2. *Aujeszky diseases virus (ADV)*

The ADV is the target of numerous control and eradication programs, and many of those programs have already achieved success and the aujeszky-free status. The ADV is the causative agent of the Aujeszky disease (AD), that is characterized by clinical respiratory signs and nervous and serious reproductive disorders [50].

The ADV had been isolated from prepuce and detected in the semen of the reproducers [51]. In 1984, [52] carried out a study with experimental infections. They observed that testicular degeneration and decreased semen quality due to fever of the infected animals are frequent in ADV-positive animals.

The DA suspicion is raised by symptoms, but laboratory tests are necessary for the definitive diagnosis, since the virus can be detected in tissues or secretions of the animals through virological diagnosis. Serologic tests can be used, and ELISA is the most indicated because it can differentiate the antibodies proceeding from the immune response of the vaccines with antigenic markers from those ones infected with the field virus [53].

Eradication through vaccination, removal of the infected animals and depopulation of the positive farms have achieved success in several countries [54]. However, care must be taken with the wild pigs which are PRV reservoirs [55].

3.2.3. Classical swine fever virus (CSFV)

The virus of the classical swine fever belongs to Pestvirus genus. It is highly contagious and causes the classical swine fever (CSF), with mortality rates ranging from 80 to 90% and leads to a framework of generalized bleedings. The contact with wild animals and infected food and the transit of animals are the main forms for CSFV dissemination. Therefore, the marketing of semen for AI is considered an additional hazard [56].

In an experimental study, van Rijn et al [57] (2004) observed the presence of CSFV in pigs' semen at 3 days after infection. The elimination continued intermittently until the end of the experiment (18 days), as proving that artificial insemination can be a risk factor for transmission of the disease.

Due to importance of the disease, the clinical suspicion should be investigated by laboratory techniques. While virus isolation is the gold standard, other tests such as ELISA and RT-PCR can be used for definitive diagnosis [58, 59]. The tonsils, spleen, pharyngeal and mesenteric ganglions are the favorite organs for sending to laboratories.

In the case of diagnostic confirmation, several procedures should be taken in order to prevent the virus from spreading through the region. The sacrifice of the positive animals, the prohibition that animals and semen to transit in the region as well as the installation of sanitary barriers are actions for controlling the outbreak. Another control procedure is vaccination, however only attenuated alive vaccines are available, as hampering the differentiation between vaccinated and infected animals [60].

3.2.4. African Swine Fever Virus (ASFV)

The African swine fever virus is the causative agent of the african swine fever (ASF), that is a highly contagious and lethal disease characterized by a clinical picture similar to that of the classical swine fever [61, 62]. The epidemiological characteristics of the disease include the potential for rapid dissemination through direct and indirect contact as well as a natural transmission via arthropods and wild Suidae.

The virus of the African swine fever was isolated from the semen of infected pigs [6, 57]. The virus elimination through bodily secretions can last up to 70 days in persistently infected animals [63], which are the main villain in dissemination of the virus in herd.

Besides the epidemiological importance, the persistently infected animals are the major obstacle to diagnosis because they present less severe clinical signs, as requiring confidential laboratory tests in order to establish a reliable definitive diagnosis of ASF as well as to provide relevant information about the time of infection in order to successfully support the control and eradication programs [64]. The viral isolation is an important tool for diagnosis, however it is a laborious and very slow procedure. The PCR technique has good sensitivity and specificity and is a faster alternative for detection of the virus [61].

Because of the unavailability of the vaccine against ASFV, the control strategies involve circulation restrictions, biosecurity and stamping out [65]. In Spain, the successful ASF eradication has been associated with the screening and removal of the persistently infected pigs [66].

3.2.5. *Porcine circovirus 2*

The *porcine circovirus 2* (PCV2) is the causative agent of the porcine circovirosis and may present six different clinical syndromes, that are the multisystemic weakening syndrome (PMWS), dermatitis and nephropathy syndrome, the reproductive, respiratory, digestive and nervous failures [67, 68]. However, PMWS and the reproductive failures are only ones caused by PCV2 without the presence of cofactors [69].

In the aborted, stillbirths and/or mummified fetuses, the inflammatory changes can be observed in the myocardium associated with depletion of lymphoid tissues [69]. In those situations, the probable infection source of the females is the contamination of the positive male' semen. Opriessnig et al. [70] (2006) demonstrated through IHC the presence of the virus in cells of the testis, epididymis and accessory glands.

Besides IHC, the PCV2 can be detected by hybridization in situ (HIS) and PCR [71]. The virus isolation can also be used. However, the virus produces no cytopathic effect in the cells, therefore it is necessary to detect the viral antigen by immunofluorescence or immunochemistry.

Recently, Blomqvist et al. [72] evaluated the reduction of the viral load in semen after single layer centrifugation followed by a swim-up. They observed a reduction higher than 99% in the semen samples. Furthermore, the commercial vaccines have been very effective for controlling the disease in infected herd.

3.2.6. *Porcine parvovirus*

The porcine parvovirus (PPV) has worldwide distribution and is responsible for reproductive failures that are characterized by embryonic death, fetal mummification and stillbirth [73]. PPV can be a non encapsulated virus. It is resistant to adverse environmental conditions, which facilitates its dissemination. In addition, there may be venereal transmission of the virus from the infected semen. Besides the semen, the virus can be detected in testis, in the scrotal lymph nodes and in epididymis [6].

The techniques for virus detection are diverse and the direct immunofluorescence and PCR are the most commonly used methods. Serology can also confirm the presence of the anti-PPV antibodies. Although the virus isolation may be necessary to detect the viral sample, the fetal tissues are toxic to cellular cultures, therefore limiting the use of this technique in some situations [74].

The PPV-induced reproductive failures can be prevented by making sure that the development of the females' immune response occurred before conception. The immune response can result from natural exposure or from vaccination which is a common practice and performed at least annually [74].

4. The interference of diseases in AI efficiency

In swine, the efficiency of the AI programs is related to higher pregnancy rates, reduced estrus repetition rates and high number of the piglets born per litter. However, to obtain reproductive efficiency, several parameters must be optimized such as the animal nutrition, thermal comfort, skilled labor, genetics and mainly the sanitary aspect. This last factor is fundamental for the herd of the animals involved in reproduction to be totally free from disease and properly immunized against the most common diseases that can lead to reproductive disorders.

Therefore, the assurance of the animals' health is extremely important to ensure the absence of contamination of the animals' semen. From the scientific evidence that the presence of a virus or bacteria in the male' semen may reduce the fertility rates in the male and the female to be inseminated, the animal contamination by infectious diseases should be avoided.

The direct impact that occurs in males is mainly related to reduction in the sperm quality and numbers of doses produced. The reason for the impairment of the semen quality is not totally elucidated. Therefore, the losses to the farmer is considerable because it is often necessary to discard the boar because irreversible degenerative changes at testicular and epididymal levels by diseases that lead to fever for prolonged periods.

Solis et al. [75] reported that the experimental infection of the animals with porcine rubulavirus (PoRV), which causes the blue eye disease (BED) was able to cause orchitis in animals, as also affecting the portion of the epididymis. The virus was detected in the semen, either in the sperm and jell fraction. Those researchers observed the ability of this virus to cause severe alterations in sperm concentration, motility and morphology of the infected animals'. Those changes were aggravated according to the time of the sperm storage. Taking into account that the virus does not affect the adjacent glands, the seminal volume remained unchanged. The changes in other parameters occurred due to inflammatory event of the virus on the spermatic ducts, as leading to loss of the spermatic cells. Most viruses behave like aforementioned, however there are still many doubts about the extent of the virus interaction with the spermatozoids. Thus, future molecular studies are needed to elucidate the mechanism of those diseases.

In females, reports suggest that PRRSV was previously isolated from ovaries of infected animals, particularly locating in either granulose cells layer and theca cells layer in atretic follicles of those animals. However, there are no reports of this virus in sows' oocytes [76, 77] neither the viral effect on their development ability. In infections associated with PCV 2, the oocytes collected from serum-positive animals for infection did not show to be positive for

http://dx.doi.org/10.5772/52337

the presence of the virus. Thus, the contamination via oocytes in naturally infected animals is not a natural route [78]. Yet this author and collaborators found that the virus can adhere firmly to either oocyte-cumulus complex and pellucid zone of embryos at the initial development stage despite not affecting the embryonic development.

At embryonic level, it has been demonstrated that the replication of some viruses can occur in the embryonic cells. In this context, the Pellucid Zone (ZP) of the embryos acts as a barrier protecting the embryo against viral agents. Therefore, after disruption of the pellucid zone at stage of the hatched blastocysts, some viruses such as the classical swine fever virus and PCV-2 can replicate in embryonic cells as carrying a deleterious effect, especially in embryos produced in vitro [79, 80]. The greatest weakness of the embryos produced in vitro may be due either to a thinner pellucid zone of those embryos [81] and greater exposure to laboratorial conditions and culture media that can act as contamination sources. It is known that ZP of pig embryos is much stickier than that of cattle, although the reason for this fact to be not known [82]. It is believed that lower-sized virus (20 -26 nm), such as *porcine circovirus 2* and porcine parvovirus could even surpass the ZP of embryos produced in vivo by promoting contamination of the embryonic cells [13, 80]. However, this issue is still controversial and further studies are still needed.

Thus, it is expected the contamination of the embryonic cells of the ZP-unprovided embryos will depend mainly on nature of the virus, of the embryonic development stage and the presence of viral receptors expressed in target cells [82]. Furthermore, the ZP- unprovided embryos that are produced in vitro are much more sensitive to viral contamination and, independent of the nature, they represent a real source for contamination of the animals mainly by diseases caused by virus. Finally, the disinfection of the swine embryos by using washing and treatment with enzymatic combination rather represents a reasonable alternative for programs of the in vitro embryonic production [78].

5. Possible control procedure to be performed

Because the differences in the prevalence rates of the diseases among countries and even regions, the control strategies will differ according to incidence of each disease. Therefore, the policies for eradication, vaccination and isolation of the animals in farms are very dependable on the types of disease the animals would be more exposed.

The preventive procedures against transmission of infectious diseases via semen depend on the control routine. The AI must be understood as a contaminative potential for swine females, since it is a vehicle for disease transmission. Thus, the insemination centers should be regularly controlled and monitored according to specific criteria. However, even before considering the potential for contamination through semen, it is necessary to pay attention to the possibility for disease introduction through acquisition of a living animal. Thus, some practices such as the introduction of animals which are serologically negative or animals proceeding from seronegative herds and to avoid the contact of the animals pertaining to insemination center with external people are essential to prevent the introduction of diseases. After acquisition and routinely on farms, the male considered as potential disease disseminator only will be introduced in the semen collect program after a quarantine period, during which he remains isolated and under observation in order to verify if there is any abnormality sign. After introduction of the male in the breeding herds, it should be daily observed for signs indicating clinical disease. In the case of any abnormality in those animals, semen collections should be immediately interrupted. This method is highly effective for controlling the diseases that present evident clinical signs.

Diseases that have high dissemination potential and can be transmitted via aerosols, such as PRRS and AD, as might cause high losses in the farms should be monitored through periodic serological tests. Another important factor to be considered is the hygiene in the farm. The cleaning and disinfection of the installations before the entry of the animals, besides respecting the sanitary break period, are essential to prevent the dissemination of the pathogens.

The effective use of the antimicrobials to control contamination in diluents can act effectively, as minimizing the action of the bacterial and fungal agents [82]. Currently, there are many antimicrobial agents commonly used in seminal diluents such as aminocyclitols, aminoglycosides, beta-lactams, lincosamides and macrolides. However, these agents do not prove to be totally effective against some of the disease causing agents [18]. In routine of the farm, the antibiotics are added to seminal portions, as expecting high level of accidental contamination in the attempt to reduce the proliferation of bacteria.

Although the availability of the studies including the use of the antiviral drugs to inhibit the replication of the virus in the male's reproductive tract [83], the control of viral pathogens still needs to be better understood and will follow the pathway similarly to the one accomplished for bacteria [5]. Unlike the semen treatment with antibiotics, which can reduce or prevent the dissemination of venereal diseases caused by bacteria, the antiviral agents used to prevent contamination of the semen are not adopted in the swine IA industry. Therefore, many countries have adopted other successful strategies in maintenance of the specific viral pathogen-free centers. In those centers, the main control strategies are based on animal monitoring program for specific viruses. The animals are serologically evaluated and the serologically positive animals are readily eliminated from breeding herds [6].

As previously mentioned, recently Blomqvist et al. [72] observed a reduction higher than 99% at PCV2 concentration in semen samples. This new technique has shown to be effective against several other viral agents, which are present in samples of the human semen and other domestic species' [84-87]. Thus, this method represents a promising alternative for the control of viral contamination in the pigs' semen.

Another possibility for controlling the dissemination of diseases would be the programs for vaccination against the main agents that can be carried by semen and lead to diseases in

http://dx.doi.org/10.5772/52337

sow. However, there is no vaccine against some of those agents such as the ASF case, therefore making necessary the individual control methods as previously detailed.

6. Conclusion

The increasing tendency of the international trade in pigs' embryos and gametes has been stimulating an intensive investigation of the disease transmission via semen and porcine embryos. There are numerous diseases, both bacterial and viral causes, which are linked to transmission via boars' semen. In particular, each agent provides a type of interaction with gametes and has a specific site of action, which hinders the establishment of specific control procedures. Thus, despite the promising researches, many conclusive studies are required to ensure the innocuousness of the gametes from the infected animals. In addition, the effective and rapid diagnostic methods and effective control procedures should be developed and optimized in order to allow the access to swine farmers.

Acknowledgments

The autors thank the book editor Dr. Alemayehu Lemma for comments, Ms. Iva Simic by the invitation and Federal University of Viçosa for the financial support.

Author details

Emílio César Martins Pereira[1,2*], Abelardo Silva Júnior[3], Eduardo Paulino da Costa[4] and Carlos Eduardo Real Pereira[5]

*Address all correspondence to: emiliovet2004@hotmail.com

1 Animal Reproduction Laboratory, Faculty of Veterinary Medicine and Zootechny, São Paulo State University, Botucatu, Brazil

2 Institute of Agricultural Sciences, Federal University of Viçosa, Rio Paranaíba, Brazil

3 Animal Virology Laboratory, Veterinary Department, Federal University of Viçosa, Viçosa, Brazil

4 Animal Reproduction Laboratory, Veterinary Department, Federal University of Viçosa, Viçosa, Brazil

5 Animal Pathology Laboratory, Department of Veterinary, Federal University of Minas Gerais, Belo Horizonte, Brazil

References

[1] ABIPECS 2012 http://www.abipecs.org.br/pt/estatisticas/mundial/producao-2.html (acessed 2 June 2012)

[2] Gerrits R.J., Lunney J.K., Johnson L.A., Pursel, V.G., Kraeling R.R., Rohrer G.A., Dobrinsky J.R. Perspectives for artificial insemination and genomics to improve global swine populations. Theriogenology. 2005;63 283 – 299.

[3] Riesenbeck A. Review on International Trade with Boar Semen. Reproduction in Domestic Animals. 2011;46(2) 1–3.

[4] Feitsma R. Artificial insemination in pigs, research and developments in The Netherlands, a review. Acta Scientiae Veterinariae, 2009;37(1) 61-71.

[5] Althouse G.C., Rossow K. The Potential Risk of Infectious Disease Dissemination Via Artificial Insemination in Swine. Reproduction in Domestic Animals. 2011;46(2) 64–67.

[6] Guérin B., Pozzi N. Viruses in boar semen: detection and clinical as well as epidemiological consequences regarding disease transmission by artificial insemination. Theriogenology. 2005;63 556-572.

[7] Romero C.H., Meade P.N., Shultz J.E., Chung H.Y., Gibbs E.P., Hahn E.C., Lollis G. Venereal transmission of pseudorabies viruses indigenous to feral swine. Journal of Wildlife Diseases. 2001;37(2) 289–296.

[8] Oliveria S.J., Wesley I.V., Baetz A.L., Harmon K.M., Kader I.I.T.A., Uzeda M. Arcobacter cryaerophilus and Arcobacter butzleri isolated from preputial fluid of boars and fattening pigs in Brazil. Jornal Veterinary Diagnostic Investigation. 1999;11 462–464.

[9] Osorio F.A. Latency of Aujeszky's disease virus. Veterinary Research. 2000;31 117-118.

[10] Madson D.M., Patterson A.R., Ramamoorthy S., Pal, N., Meng X.J., Opriessnig T. Reproductive Failure Experimentally Induced in Sows via Artificial Insemination with Semen Spiked with Porcine Circovirus Type 2. Veterinary Pathology. 2009;46 707–716.

[11] Langfeldt N., Wendt M., Amtsberg G. Comparative studies of the detection of Corynebacterium suis infections in swine by indirect immunofluorescence and culture. Berl Munch Tierarztl Wochenschr. 1990;103 273-276.

[12] Christopher-Hennings J., Nelson E.A., Hines R.J., Nelson J.K., Swenson S.L., Zimmerman J.J., Chase C.L., Yaeger M.J., Benfield D.A. Persistence of porcine reproductive and respiratory syndrome virus in serum and semen of adult boars. Journal of Veterinary Diagnostic Investigation. 1995;7 456-64.

[13] Althouse G.C. Sanitary procedures for the production of extended semen. Reproduction in Domestic Animals. 2008;43 374–378.

[14] Madec F., Albina E., Vannier P. Les agents infectieux dans le sperme de verrat. Association Française de Medecine Veterinaire Porcine. AFMPP, Maisons-Alfort, France 1994 150.

[15] Larsen R.E., Shope R.E.J., Leman A.D., Kurtz H.J. Semen changes in boars after experimental infection with pseudorabies virus. American Journal Veterninary Research. 1980;41 733-39.

[16] Sone, M. Investigations on the control of bacteria in boar semen. Japanese Journal of Animal Reproduction. 1990;36 23–29.

[17] Althouse G., Kuster C., Clark S., Weisiger R. Field investigations of bacterial contaminants and their effects on extended porcine semen. Theriogenology. 2000;53 1167–1176.

[18] Althouse G., Lu, K. Bacteriospermia in extended porcine semen. Theriogenology, 2005;63 573–584.

[19] Maes D., Nauwynck H., Rijsselaere T., Mateusen B., Vyt P., de Kruif A., Van Soom A. Diseases in swine transmitted by artificial insemination: An overview. Theriogenology. 2008;70 1337–1345.

[20] Favero A.C.M., Pinheiro S.R., Vasconcellos S.A., Morais Z.M., Ferreira F., Ferreira Neto J.S. Most frequent serovars of leptospires in serological tests of buffaloes, sheeps, goats, horses, swines and dogs from several Brazilian states. Ciencia Rural 2002;32 613–619.

[21] Boqvist S., Thu H.T.V, Vagsholm I., Magnusson U. The impact of Leptospira seropositivity on reproductive performance in sows in southern Viet Nam.Theriogenology 2002;58 1327–35.

[22] Adler B., de la Penã Moctezuma A. Leptospira and leptospirosis. Veterinary Microbiology. 2010;140 287–296.

[23] Adler B., Lo M., Seemann T., Murray G. L. Pathogenesis of leptospirosis: The influence of genomics. Veterinary Microbiology. 2011;153 73-81.

[24] Ellis W.A. Diagnosis of leptospirosis in farm animals. In The Present State of Leptospirosis Diagnosis and Control. Dordrecht,Boston, Lancaster, Martinus Nijhoff.1986; 13-31.

[25] Maestrone G. The use of an improved fluorescent anti- body procedure in the demonstration of leptospira in animal tissues. Canadian Journal of Comparative Medicine and Veterinary Science. 1963;27 108-112.

[26] Guimarães, M.C. Epidemiologia e controle da leptospirose bovina. Importância do portador renal e do seu controle terapêutico. Comunidade Científica da Faculdade de Medicina Veterinária e Zootecnia. 1983;6 21–34.

[27] Mijs W., de Haas P., Rossau R., Van der Laan T., Rigouts L., Portaels F., van Soolingen D. Molecular evidence to support a proposal to reserve the designation Mycobacterium avium subsp. avium for birdtype isolates and M. avium subsp. hominissuis for the human/porcine type of M. avium. International Journal Systematic and Evolutionary Microbiology. 2002;52 1505–1518.

[28] Ellsworth S.R., Kirkbride C.A., Johnson D.D., Vorhies M.W. Mycobacterium avium abortion in a sow. Veterinary Pathology. 1979;16 310–317.

[29] Wellenberg G.J., de Haas P.E., van Ingen J., van Soolingen D., Visser I.J. Multiple strains of Mycobacterium avium subspecies hominissuis infections associated with aborted fetuses and wasting in pigs. Veterinary Record. 2010;167 451–454.

[30] Eisenberg T., Volmer R., Eskens U., Moser I., Nesseler A., Sauerwald C., Seeger H., Klewer-Fromenti, K., Mobius P. Outbreak of reproductive disorders and mycobacteriosis in swine associated with a single strain of Mycobacterium avium subspecies hominissuis. Veterinary. Microbiology. 2012. In press (accessed 12 June 2012). http://www.sciencedirect.com/science/article/pii/S0378113512001800

[31] Domingos M., Amado A., Botelho A. IS1245 RFLP analysis of strains of Mycobacterium avium subspecies hominissuis isolated from pigs with tuberculosis lymphadenitis in Portugal.Veterinary Record. 2009;164 116-120.

[32] Alvarez J., Castellanos E., Romero B., Aranaz A., Bezos J. Epidemiological investigation of a Mycobacterium avium subsp. hominissuis outbreak in swine. Epidemiology and Infection. 2011;139 143-148.

[33] Pakarinen J., Nieminen T., Tirkkonen T., Tsitko I., Ali-Vehmas T., Neubauer P., Salkinoja-Salonen M.S.. Proliferation of mycobacteria in a piggery environment revealed by Mycobacterium-specific realtime quantitative PCR and 16S rRNA sandwich hybridization. Veterinary Microbiology. 2007;120 105–112.

[34] Godfroid J., Cloeckaer, A., Liautard J.P., Kohler S., Fretin D., Walravens K., Garin-Bastuji B., Letesson J.J. From the discovery of the Malta fever's agent to the discovery of a marine mammal reservoir, brucellosis has continuously been a re-emerging zoonosis. Veterinary Research. 2005;36 313–326.

[35] Liautard J.P., Gross A., Dornand J., Kohler S. Interactions between professional phagocytes and Brucela sp. Microbiologia. 1996;12 196-206.

[36] Fayazi Z., Ghadersohi A., Hirst R.G. Development of a Brucella suis specific hybridisation probe and PCR which distinguishes B. suis from Brucella abortus. Veterinary Microbiology. 2002;84 253-261.

[37] Kauffold J., Melzer F., Henning K., Schulze K., Leiding C., Sachse K. Prevalence of chlamydiae in boars and semen used forartificial insemination. Theriogenology 2006;65 1750–1758.

[38] Busch M., Thoma R., Schiller I., Corboz L., Pospischil A. Occurrence of chlamydiae in the genital tracts of sows at slaughter and their possible significance for reproductive failure. Journal of Veterinary Medicine B. 2000;47 471–480.

[39] Schautteet K., Vanrompay, D. Chlamydiaceae infections in pig. Veterinary Research. 2011;42 29.

[40] Schiller, I., Koesters R., Weilenmann R., Kaltenboeck B., Pospischil A. Polymerase chain reaction (PCR) detection of porcine Chlamydia trachomatis and Ruminant C. psittaciserovar 1 DNA in formalin-fixed intestinal specimens from swine. Journal of Veterinary Medicine B. 1997;44 185–191.

[41] Land J.A., Van Bergen J.E.A.M., Morre S.A., Postma M.J. Epidemiology of Chlamydia trachomatis infection in women and the cost-effectiveness of screening. Human Reproduction Update 2010;16 189–204.

[42] Prieto C., Castro J. Porcine reproductive and respiratory syndrome virus infection in the boar: a review. Theriogenology. 2005;63 1–16.

[43] Christopher-Hennings J., Holler L., Benfield D., Nelson E. Detection and duration of porcine reproductive and respiratory syndrome virus in semen, serum, peripheral blood mononuclear cells, and tissues from Yorkshire, Hampshire and Landrace boars. Journal of Veterinary Diagnostic Investigation. 2001;13 133–142.

[44] Feitsma H., Grooten H., van Schie F., Colenbrander B. 12th international congress on animal reproduction Conference Proceedings, 1992. The effect of porcine epidemic abortion and respiratory syndrome (PEARS) on sperm production. The Hague.

[45] Christopher-Hennings J., Nelson E., Nelson J., Benfield D. Effects of a modified-live vaccine against porcine reproductive and respiratory syndrome virus in boars. American Journal of Veterinary Research. 1997;58 40–45.

[46] Kim H.S., Kwang J., Yoon I.J., Joo H.S., Frey M.L. Enhanced replication of porcine reproductive and respiratory syndrome (PRRS) virus in a homogeneous subpopulation of MA-104 cell line. Archieves of Virology. 1993;133 477-483.

[47] Magar R., Larochelle R., Robinson Y., Dubuc, C. Immunohistochemical detection of porcine reproductive and respiratory syndrome virus using colloidal gold. Canadian Journal of Veterinary Research. 1993;57 300-304.

[48] Suarez P., Zardoya R., Prieto C., Solana A., Tabares E., Bautista J.M., Castro J.M. Direct detection of the porcine reproductive and respiratory syndrome (PRRS) virus by reverse polymerase chain-reaction (RT-PCR). Archieves of Virology. 1994;135 89-99.

[49] Linhares D.C.L., Cano J.P., Wetzell T., Neremc J., Torremorell M., Dee S.A. Effect of modified-live porcine reproductive and respiratory syndrome virus (PRRSv) vaccine

on the shedding of wild-type virus from an infected population of growing pigs. Vaccine. 2012;30 407-413.

[50] Pomeranz L.E., Reynolds A.E., Hengartner C.J. Molecular biology of pseudorabies virus: impact on neurovirology and veterinary medicine. Microbiology and Molecular Biology Reviews. 2005;69(3) 462–500.

[51] Medveczky I., Szabo I. Isolation of Aujeszky's disease virus from boar semen. Acta Veterinaria Academiae Scientiarum Hungaricae. 1981;29 29-35.

[52] Hall L.B.Jr., Kluge J.P., Evans L-E., Clark T-L; Hill H.J. Testicular changes observed in boars following experimental inoculation with pseudorabies Aujeszky's virus. Canadian Journal of Comparative Medicine. 1984;48 303-307.

[53] Serena M.S., Metz G.E., Corva S.G., Mórtola E.C., Echeverría M.G. A differential ELISA based on recombinant immunodominant epitopes of the gE gene of SHV-1 in a baculovirus–insect cell system to discriminate between pigs infected naturally with pseudorabies and vaccinated pigs. Journal of Virological Methods. 2011;171 388-393.

[54] Boadella M., Gortazar C., Vicente J., Ruiz-Fons F. Wild boar: an increasing concern for Aujeszky's disease control in pigs? BMC Veterinary Research. 2012;8 7.

[55] Hahn E.C., Bahaa F-A., Lichtensteiger C.A. Variation of Aujeszky's disease viruses in wild swine in USA. Veterinary Microbiology. 2010;143 45-51.

[56] Floegel G., Wehrendc A., Depnera K.R., Fritzemeierb J., Waberskic D., Moennig V. Detection of Classical Swine Fever virus in semen of infected boars. Veterinary Microbiology. 2000;77 109-116.

[57] Van Rijn P.A., Wellenberg G.J., Van der Honing R.H., Jacobs L., Moonena P.L.J.M., Feitsma H. Detection of economically important viruses in boar semen by quantitative RealTime PCR technology. Journal of virological methods. 2004;120 151-160.

[58] Dewulf J., Koenen F., Mintiens K., Denis P., Ribbens S., Kruif A. Analytical performance of several classical swine fever laboratory diagnostic techniques on live animals for detection of infection. Journal of virological methods. 2004;119 137-143.

[59] Fosgate G.T., Tavompanich S., Hunter D., Pugh R., Sterle J.A, Schumann K.R., Eberling A.J., Beckham T.R., Martin B.M., Clarke N.P., Adams L.G. Diagnostic specificity of a real-time RT-PCR in cattle for foot-and-mouth disease and swine for foot-and-mouth disease and classical swine fever based on non-invasive specimen collection. Veterinary Microbiology. 2008;132 158-164.

[60] Van Oirschot J.T. Vaccinology of classical swine fever: from lab to field. Veterinary Microbiology. 2003;96 367-384.

[61] Tignon M., Gallardo C., Iscaroc C., Hutetd E., Van der Stedee Y., Kolbasovf D., De Mia G.M., Le Potierd M.F., Bishopg R.P., Ariasb M., Koenene, F. Development and inter-laboratory validation study of an improved new real-time PCR assay with in-

ternal control for detection and laboratory diagnosis of African swine fever virus. Journal of Virological Methods. 2011;178 161-170.

[62] Kleiboeker S.B. Swine fever: classical swine fever and African swine fever. Veterinary Clinics of North America: Food Animal Practice. 2002;18 431–451.

[63] Carvalho Ferreira H.C., Weesendorp E., Elbers A.R.W., Bouma A., Quak S., Stegeman J.A., Loeffen W.L.A. African swine fever virus excretion patterns in persistently infected animals: A quantitative approach. Veterinary Microbiology.2012; [Epub ahead of print].

[64] OIE, 2008. Chapter 2.8.1. African swine fever. In: Manual of Diagnostic Tests and Vaccines for Terrestrial Animals 2008. Office International des Epizooties, Paris, France.

[65] OIE, 2011. Terrestrial Animal Health Code. World Organisation for Animal Health, Paris, France.

[66] Arias M., Sanchez-Vizcaino J.M. Trends in Emerging Viral Infections of Swine. Iowa. Iowa State University Press. 2002.

[67] Opriessnig T., Meng X.-J., Halbur P.G. Porcine circovirus type 2-associated disease: Update on current terminology, clinical manifestations, pathogenesis, diagnosis, and intervention strategies. Journal of Veterinary Diagnostic Investigation. 2007;19 591–615.

[68] Chae C. A review of porcine circovirus 2-associated syndromes and diseases. Veterinary Journal. 2005;169(3) 326-336.

[69] Allan G.M., McNeilly F. 19th International Pig Veterinary Society. Congress. 2006. PMWS/PCVD, Diagnosis, disease and control: what do we know? Copenhagen.

[70] Opriessnig T., Kuster C., Halbur P.G. Demonstration of porcine circovirus type 2 in the testes and accessory sex glands of a boar. Journal of Swine Health Production. 2006;14 42–45.

[71] Segales, J. Porcine circovirus type 2 (PCV2) infections: Clinical signs, pathology and laboratory diagnosis. Virus Reserarch. 2012;164 10-19.

[72] Blomqvist G., Perssona M., Wallgrenb M., Wallgrena P., Morrellc J.M. Removal of virus from boar semen spiked with porcine circovirus type 2. Animal Reproduction Science. 2011;126 108-114.

[73] Mengeling W.L., Paul P.S., Brown T.T. Transplacental infection and embryonic death following maternal exposure to PPV near time of conception. Archives of Virology. 1980;65 645–652.

[74] Mengeling W.L., Lager K.M., Vorwald A.C. The effect of porcine parvovirus and porcine reproductive and respiratory syndrome virus on porcine reproductive performance. Animal Reproduction Science. 2000;60-61 199-210.

[75] Solís M., Ramírez-Mendoza H., Mercado C., Espinosa S., Vallejo V., Reyes-Leyva J., Hernández J. Semen alterations in porcine rubulavirus-infected boars are related to viral excretion and have implications for artificial insemination. Research in Veterinary Science. 2007;83 403–409.

[76] Gregg K., Xiang T., Arenivas S.S., Hwang E., Arenivas F., Chen S.H., Walker S., Picou A., Polejaeva I. Risk assessment of porcine reproductive and respiratory syndrome virus (PRRSV) transmission via somatic cell nuclear transfer (SCNT) embryo production using oocytes from commercial abattoirs. Animal Reproduction Science. 2011;125 148-157.

[77] Sur J.H., Doster A.R., Galeota J.A., Osorio F.A. Evidence for the localization of porcine reproductive and respiratory syndrome virus (PRRSV) antigen and RNA in ovarian follicles in gilts. Veterinary Pathology. 2001;38 58–66.

[78] Bielanski A., Larochelle R., Magar R. An attempt to render oocytes and embryos free from the porcine circovirus type 2 after experimental in vitro exposure. Canadian Journal of Veterinary Research. 2004;68 222-225.

[79] Mateusen B., Sanchez R.E., Van Soom A., Meerts P., Maes D.G., Nauwynck H.J. Susceptibility of pig embryos to porcine circovirus type 2 infection. Theriogenology. 2004;61 91–101.

[80] Schüürmann E., Flögel-Niesmann G., Mönnig V., Rath D. Susceptibility of in vivo- and in vitro-produced porcine embryos to classical swine fever virus. Reproduction in Domestic Animals. 2005;40 415-421.

[81] Funahashi H., Ekwall H., Rodriguez-Martinez H. Zona reaction in porcine oocytes fertilized in vivo and in vitro as seen with scanning electron microscopy. Biology of Reproduction. 2000;63 1437–1442.

[82] van Soom A., Wrathall A.E., Herrler A., Nauwynck H.J. Is the zona pellucida an efficient barrier to viral infection? Reproduction, Fertility and Development. 2010;22 21-31.

[83] Christopher-Hennings J., Nelson E.A., Althouse G.C., Lunney J. Comparative antiviral and proviral factors in semen and vaccines for preventing viral dissemination from the male reproductive tract and semen. Animal Health Research Reviews. 2008;9 59–69.

[84] Bujan L., Daudin M., Alvarez M., Massip P., Puel J., Pasquier C. Intermittent human immunodefiency type 1 virus (HIV-1) shedding in semen and efficiency of sperm processing despite high seminal HIV-1 RNA levels. Fertility and Sterility. 2002;78 1321–1323.

[85] Cassuto N.G., Sifer C., Feldmann G., Bouret D., Moret F., Benifla J.L., Porcher R., Naouri M., Neuraz A., Alvarez S., Poncelet C., Madelenat P., Devaux A. A modified RT-PCR technique to screen for viral RNA in the semen of hepatitis C virus-positive men. Human Reproduction. 2002;17 3153–3156.

[86] Levy R., Bourlet T., Maertens A., Salle B., Lomage J., Laurent J.L., Pozzetto B., Guerin J.F. Pregnancy after safe IVF with hepatitis C virus RNA-positive sperm. Human Reproduction. 2002;17 2650–2653.

[87] Morrell J.M., Geraghty R.J. Effective removal of equine arteritis virus from stallion semen. Equine Veterinary Journal. 2006;38 224–229.

Chapter 8

The Role of Trans-Rectal Ultrasonography in Artificial Insemination Program

Alemayehu Lemma

Additional information is available at the end of the chapter

http://dx.doi.org/10.5772/52721

1. Introduction

The ultrasound technology has been used for various functions particularly as a tool in beef and dairy research for many years. It has become more available to the commercial livestock agriculture recently. Application of transrectal real-time ultrasonography in the study of bovine reproduction represents a technological breakthrough that has revolutionized the knowledge of reproductive biology [Boyd and Omran, 1991]. New research results derived from ultrasonic imaging has clarified the complex nature of reproductive processes such as ovarian follicular dynamics, corpus luteum function, and foetal development in farm animals. Extensive adoption and use of ultrasonography for routine reproductive examinations of dairy cattle is its highest contribution to the dairy industry.

Practical applications of ultrasound in bovine reproduction include imaging of the ovary as a diagnostic aid, examination and confirmation of ovarian cysts, early pregnancy detection, identification of twins and foetal sexing [Fortune et al, 1988; Garcia et al, 1999; Noble et al, 2000 Lamb, 2001; Stroud, 2006]. Although rectal palpation is the established method for conducting reproductive examinations, the information-gathering capabilities of ultrasonic imaging far exceed those of rectal palpation. Assessment of pregnancy status and foetal viability early post breeding can significantly improve reproductive efficiency. Such methods can play a key role in reproductive management to rapidly return open animals to the breeding program. Early pregnancy detection is only useful when techniques have a high level of accuracy for detection of both pregnant and non-pregnant animals.

Early ultrasonic identification of twinning or male calves in dairy cows allows for implementation of differential management strategies such as termination of the unwanted pregnancy or to mitigate the negative effects of twinning during the periparturient period. Ultrasound can accurately determine the presence of a viable embryo as early as 21 days after AI. The accuracy of detecting foetal viability may approach 100% [Lamb, 2001]. A technician with a trained eye has the capability of accurately assessing the age of the foetus based on foetal size [Curran, 1986]. At 60 to 85 days of pregnancy the trained user can even determine foetal sex by the absence and/or presence of the foetal genitalia with over 95% accuracy. These two features alone provide many options for the use of ultrasound in reproductive management practices [Palmer and Drinacourt, 1980; Muller and Wittkowski, 1986; Kastelic et al, 1989; Romano and Masgee, 2001]. Development of integrated reproductive management systems that combines ultrasound with new and existing reproductive technologies will further enhance the practical applications of ultrasonography. In summary, current and future applications of ultrasonography hold tremendous potential to enhance reproductive management and improve reproductive efficiency in bovine.

The incorporation of ultrasound in reproductive research has also led to greater understanding of ovarian physiology. Ultrasound has been used extensively in the development of controlled breeding programs involving both oestrus and ovulation synchronization for effective timed AI. Sequential monitoring of dynamic changes in a follicular population during the oestrous cycle has been made possible by ultrasonography [Driancort et al, 1991; Garcia et al, 1999; Ginther 1993]. This capability has helped unlock some of the mysteries of folliculogenesis. During anoestrous, inactive ovaries are readily differentiated from functional ovaries with ultrasonography.

Further, when choosing bulls, many producers are faced with difficult decisions regarding the contributions of both maternal and carcass traits. Not only do the attributes of multiple breeds vary, but variation within breed is also substantial. By combining ultrasound and AI, a producer can develop a breeding program that optimizes both maternal and carcass traits [Travene et al, 1985; Kahn, 1992]. Using ultrasound, producers may determine females that are pregnant with AI-sired heifer calves based on the age and sex of the foetus [Travene et al, 1985; Kahn, 1992]. In a typical commercial cow-calf production environment controlled breeding seasons range from 60 to 120 days. By using ultrasound as early as 30 days after the end of the breeding season in seasonally breeding animals, producers can divide their herd into cows that became pregnant early or late in the breeding season, and open cows which can subsequently be managed appropriately in accordance with their reproductive status to run the production at reasonable cost.

2. Evaluation of the ovaries during AI

Ultrasonic evaluation of the ovaries should be considered a routine part of the reproductive examination particularly in cattle. A 5MHz transducer has greater resolution and is more suitable for evaluation of the ovaries than a 3 or 3.5MHz transducer. Follicles, like other fluid structures, are non echogenic, and therefore, appear on the ultrasound image as black, circumscribed structures which are spherical to irregular in shape (Fig 1). The irregular shapes are attributable to compression by adjacent follicles and luteal structures of the ovarian stroma.

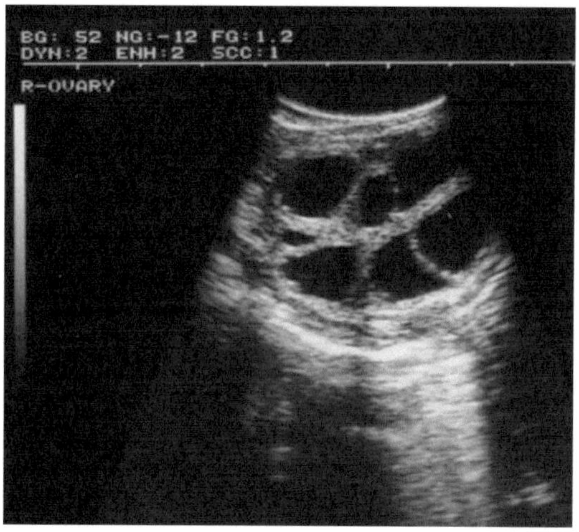

Figure 1. Several medium sized follicles observed in mare. Ultrasonogram taken with 5MHz curvilinear array scanner (Hitachi 405, Germany). Source: Lemma et al, 2006

Follicles as small as 2 - 3 mm can be seen and the corpus luteum can usually be identified throughout its functional life [Lemma et al, 2006] Estimating the stage of oestrous cycle, assessing the status and number of preovulatory follicles, determining ovulation, monitoring the development and morphology of corpus luteum are among the potential applications of ultrasonographic examination of the ovaries [Fortune et al, 1988; Garcia et al, 1999; Noble et al, 2000; Evans et al, 2000; Evans, 2003]. The number and sizes of follicles on a given ovary will vary widely and are dependent on the time of year and the reproductive stage in different animals [Vandeplassche et al, 1981; Perry, 1991; Godoi et al, 2002]. Many small follicles are observed during early dieostrus and these follicles will grow larger at mid-cycle. The dominant or ovulatory follicle will develop at a rate of 1.5 to 2.5mm per day in cattle [Driancourt et al, 1988] few days before ovulation which are all easily monitored ultrasonically to determine the date of ovulation and hence subsequently fix the appropriate time for insemination. During oestrous cycles in cattle dominant follicles reach a maximum diameter of approximately 10 - 20 mm and the largest subordinate follicles reach maximum diameter of approximately 8 mm. Cows ovulate at about 12 hours after the end of the oestrus period. The time for insemination may therefore range between 6 and 24 hours prior to ovulation [Arthur, 2001; Ball and Peters, 2004]

The appearance of dominant follicles is often accompanied by an outward manifestation of behavioural oestrus. However, cows with dominant follicle that is about to ovulate do not always show overt oestrus and this is becoming one of the greatest hindrance to the success of AI. Whilst good oestrus detection does not necessarily guarantee good reproductive performance, poor oestrus detection makes poor performance hard to avoid [Arthur, 2001]. Poor oestrus manifestation and failure to detect oestrus further hinders insemination at the correct time which is an important cause of fertilization failure. Insemination very early in oestrus also causes reduced fertility; possibly due to reduced sperm survival rates before fertilization [Andrew *et al.*, 2004].

Many developing countries commonly relay on small holder dairy production system where owners cannot afford to keep a breeding bull and have to depend on AI services. The use of AI as the main method of breeding to improve performance means that the responsibility for oestrus detection falls upon the dairy owners who manage the herd [Lemma and Kebede, 2011]. In a study conducted to compare reproductive performance between farms using AI and natural service, the NSC, CCI and DALC were significantly higher ($p<0.05$) for farms using AI (2.1; 187.0 days and 185.7 days, respectively), compared to farms using natural service (1.7; 159.1 days and 154.9 days), respectively [Lemma and Kebede, 2011]. In a different study [Hansar et al, 2011] conducted to evaluate the efficiency of oestrus detection by small holder dairy owners in the success of AI and identify the role of ultrasonic evaluation of ovarian follicles before AI in improving pregnancy rate showed that ultrasonography can solve many problems of oestrus detection. In the same study, visual oestrus detection by dairy owners was assessed for validity using ultrasonic evaluation of the ovaries before AI with the following results (Table 1).

Oestrus signs	**Overall (n=60)**	**Pregnant After AI (n=18)**	**Non-Pregnant After AI (n=42)**
Bellowing [%]	60.0	61.1	59.5
Mounting others [%]	66.7	77.8	64.2
Vaginal discharge [%]	83.3	88.9	83.3
Mounting and vaginal discharge	60.6	87.5	52.0
Diameter of dominant follicle [mm]	12.9±3.4	14.7±3.3	12.1±3.37
Estrus to AI [hrs]	13.3±9.3	10.5±6.9	15.10

Table 1. Dairy cows and heifers that showed different types of oestrus signs prior to AI (n=60)

A significant difference ($p<0.05$) was observed in the mean diameter of largest follicle between the pregnant and non pregnant animals. Similarly, the duration from detection of estrus to AI was also significantly different ($P<0.05$) between successful and failed pregnancies. While none of the animals were waited until they exhibited standing estrus, the average duration to AI for animals that later became pregnant and showed both Vaginal discharge and mounting was 6.4hrs with 13.8mm average diameter of largest follicle. In contrast to this, those non pregnant animals showing both mounting and Vaginal discharge were brought to AI on average after 14.1hrs, and the average diameter of largest follicle was 9.7mm.

The mean (±SD) diameter of the largest follicle for animals showing both signs was 12.7±4.4 mm. Considering these estrus signs to be the best indicators of estrus as perceived by the dairy owners, 9, 5 and 6 animals were brought within 6 hrs, 7-14hrs and after 14hrs of heat

http://dx.doi.org/10.5772/52721

manifestation, respectively. The mean size of the follicles for the same time group of animals was 13.5±3.2mm, 13.0±4.7mm and 11.1±5.8mm, respectively. Only 39.4% were found to be fit for insemination (showing most oestrus signs, follicular diameter ≥12mm and/or were brought for AI ≤12hrs of oestrus manifestation) during the ultrasonic evaluation. However, all animals were inseminated giving a pregnancy rate of only 30.0% compared to 61.5% for the fit animals alone. It was concluded that the low conception rate, delayed time of insemination, and the difference in the size of larger follicle indicate the incompatibility of visual heat detection and optimal time of insemination. This study clearly shows two important facts: cows showing oestrus do not necessarily carry mature follicles ready for ovulation, and ultrasonic evaluation of the ovaries right before AI can significantly improve pregnancy rate by avoiding insemination of animals that are not fit for service.

Furthermore, ultrasound has also great contribution to reproductive management through estrus synchronization. By early detection of pregnancy post AI in synchronization the pitfalls of different factors involved in reducing reproductive performance could be identified and accordingly mitigated. In a study [Hamid et al, 2012] conducted to evaluate the effects of artificial estrus induction and breed, both were known to have significant effect on pregnancy rate (Table 2). Pregnancy was determined at day 26 post AI using a B-mode real time ultrasound with a 5MHz linear array transducer (Mindray, Hong Kong). The negative effect of poor nutritional management appropriate for cross breed animals, and the positive influence of estrus induction on first service pregnancy rate were identified. This information was useful in the decision making process on those animals that failed to be pregnant.

Breed	**Non oestrus induced cows**			**Oestrus induced cows**		
	N° of cows at first AI	**Pregnancy rate [%]**	**p-value**	**N° of cows at first AI**	**Pregnancy rate [%]**	**p-value**
Zebu	75	18 (24%)		62	30 (48.4%)	
Cross	10	6 (60%)	0.018	15	7 (46.7%)	0.905
Total	85	24 (28.2%)		77	37 (48.1%)	0.009

Table 2. Comparison of first service pregnancy rate between oestrus induced and non induced cows (effect of heat induction); and between breeds (zebu and Holstein cross cows)

3. Application of ultrasonography in early PD

Reproductive ultrasonography has increased the knowledge of the changes during early pregnancy in different animals. With the use of a real-time, B-mode ultrasonography and 5 MHz transducer, pregnancy can be detected as early as 9 to 12 days post AI into gestation [Pierson and Ginther, 1984; Curran et al., 1986; Boyd et al., 1988]. A thorough understanding of the ultrasonic anatomy and dynamic changes in the uterus is essential for accurate pregnancy detection. The embryo initially appears as a short line (Day 20-22), later becomes C-shaped (Day 22-30), and finally, by Day 30-32 of gestation assumes an L- shape (Fig 2). Although the embryo can first be detected between Days 19 and 24 of gestation [Curran et al., 1986], it is most practical to scan females which are expected to have embryos that are >26 days of age. The bovine foetus can be visualized beginning at day 20 post breeding and continuing throughout gestation, however, because of its size in relation to the image field of view, the foetus cannot be fully imaged after 90 days using high frequency transducers.

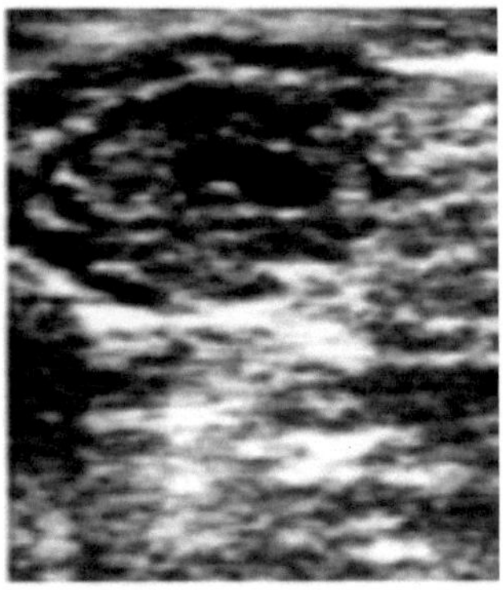

Figure 2. Bovine embryo scanned on Day 26 of pregnancy using B-mode real time ultrasound with 5MHz linear array transducer

Accuracy of diagnoses improves, however, by Day 18 (85%), Day 20 (100%) and Day 22 (100%) of pregnancy (Kastelic et al., 1989). Presence and vitality of the embryo can be confirmed by the detection of a heartbeat as early as 19 to 24 days of gestation. Early pregnancy detection has a greater economic significance particularly for the dairy industry. When an accuracy of over 99% is achieved, it enables to rapidly identify fertility problems. The rate of detection of early embryonic loss is thus also higher with 10 to 16% of cows diagnosed pregnant at 28 days post AI experience early embryonic loss by 56 days post AI. Cows diagnosed pregnant at 28 days post AI using ultrasound should, therefore, be scheduled for a subsequent examination around 60 days post AI, when the rate of embryonic loss per day decreases dramatically.

In situations where the exact dates of AI are known, ultrasonography is simply used as a confirmation of pregnancy or to validate that detection of a viable embryo within the first two weeks of pregnancy. In contrast, another study showed diagnosis of pregnancy in heifers on day 10 through day 16 of gestation resulted in a positive diagnosis for pregnant or non-pregnant cows in less than 50%. On from days 18 - 22 of gestation, accuracy of pregnancy diagnosis improved from 85% to 100% [Lamb and Fricke, 2005]. Although an embryonic vesicle is detectable by ultrasound as early as 9 days of gestation, accuracy of detection approaches 100% usually after day 25 of gestation. For practical purposes, the efficiency (speed and accuracy) of a correct diagnosis of pregnancy should be performed in cows expected to have embryos that are at least 26 days of age.

Ultrasound is a rapid method for pregnancy diagnosis, and experienced palpators adapt to ultrasound quickly. This is particularly important to lessen the effect of early scanning on embryonic survival. The time required to assess pregnancy in beef heifers at the end of a 108-day breeding season averaged 11.3 seconds using palpation per rectum versus 16.1 seconds required to assess pregnancy and foetal age using ultrasound (Galland et al., 1994). Two points must be considered when using ultrasound for routine early pregnancy diagnosis in a cow herd. First, when using ultrasound for early pregnancy diagnosis, emphasis must be given to identifying non-pregnant rather than pregnant cows. Second, a management strategy must be implemented to return the non-pregnant cows to service as quickly as possible after pregnancy diagnosis. Such strategies include administration of PGF2α to cows with a responsive CL, use of estrus detection aids, or a combination of both methods. Such strategies will significantly improve outcomes of AI in large herds.

The main advantages of the use of ultrasound for pregnancy diagnosis are the high accuracy of the results and the relatively early confirmation of pregnancy. Mistakes can be made, no matter proficient the operator might be. Therefore, it is suggested that a female not be considered non-pregnant until two negative scans have been obtained at a gestation age of at least 16 days. The main disadvantages of the use of ultrasonography are related to the cost and time involved. Ultrasound machines are relatively expensive. Pregnancy diagnosis with an ultrasound machine takes more time than rectal palpation. Also the training required for proper interpretation of the images is another disadvantage. Cows diagnosed pregnant at an early ultrasound exam have a greater risk of early embryonic loss and, therefore, must undergo subsequent pregnancy examinations to identify and rebreed cows that experience such loss. If left unidentified, cows experiencing embryonic loss after an early pregnancy diagnosis would actually reduce reproductive efficiency by extending their calving interval (Fricke, 2002).

4. Early embryonic death (EED)

Prior to the development of ultrasound for pregnancy diagnosis in cattle, veterinarians were unable to accurately determine the viability or number of embryos or foetuses. Because the heartbeat of a foetus can be detected at approximately 22 days of age, one can accurately assess whether or not the pregnancy is viable. Studies in beef [Beal et al., 1992; Lamb et al., 1997] and dairy cattle [Smith and Stevenson, 1995; Vasconcelos et al., 1997; Szenci et al., 1998] have used ultrasound to assess the incidence of embryonic loss. The fertilization rate after AI in beef cows is about 90%, whereas embryonic survival rate is 93% by day 8 and only 56% by day 12 post AI [Diskin, and Sreenan, 1980]. The incidence of embryonic loss in beef cattle appears to be significantly less than in dairy cattle. Some reports [Beal et al., 1989; 1992; Lamb and Fricke, 2005] indicate a 6.5% incidence of embryonic loss in beef cows from day 25 to day 45 of gestation. In dairy cattle, pregnancy loss from 28 to 56 days after artificial insemination may reach 13.5%, or 0.5% per day. Ultrasonography hence becomes a useful tool in the study of early embryonic death (EED), and to monitor the success of a breeding program, by determining pregnancy rates and embryonic death.

Ultrasonography also provides a tool to accurately differentiate between the failure of a female to conceive and the incidence of embryonic mortality early after AI service [Beal et al., 1989]. At present, there is no practical way to reduce early embryonic loss in lactating dairy cows. However, recognizing the occurrence and magnitude of early embryonic loss may actually present management opportunities by taking advantage of new reproductive technologies that increase AI service rate in a dairy herd. If used routinely, transrectal ultrasonography has the potential to improve reproductive efficiency within a herd by reducing the period from AI to pregnancy diagnosis to 26 to 28 days with a high degree of diagnostic accuracy [Beghelli et al, 1986; Cheffaux et al, 1986; Baxter and Ward, 1997; Meyers, 2002].

5. Conclusion

Currently fresh, chilled and frozen-thawed semen are used extensively for AI in animal breeding and production throughout the world. Dairy herd size has increased with increasing pressure to maximize milk yield, whilst at the same time reducing production costs is necessary. Accurate oestrus detection crucial for timed and successful AI and early detection of the success or otherwise of insemination can meaningfully reduce the time delay before repeated insemination if this is necessary. For these reasons it is very important to have a reliable method to accurately detect the occurrence of oestrus. Errors in efficiency and accuracy of heat detection result in high semen cost and an increase in the interval from calving to conception, reducing cow production and net returns. The use of ultrasonography prior to AI for determining the ovarian status can significantly improve the success of AI.

Conversely, reproductive management is currently a major factor affecting profitability in the dairy industry. Early identification of non-pregnant dairy cows and heifers post AI can improve reproductive efficiency and pregnancy rate by decreasing the interval between AI services and increasing AI service rate. Thus, imaging technologies such as ultrasound to identify non-pregnant dairy cows and heifers early after AI may play a key role in management strategies to improve reproductive efficiency and increase profitability on commercial and small holder dairy farms. Early detection of non-pregnancy will lead to earlier intervention and decision that will shorten the calving interval, which has economic effect on the diary farm. Transrectal ultrasonography has also been used to determine foetus viability and hence can improve the outcome of AI by allowing knowledge based decision on problem cows.

Author details

Alemayehu Lemma*

Addis Ababa University, College of Veterinary Medicine and Agriculture, Debre Zeit, Ethiopia

References

[1] Andrews, A. H., Blowey, R. W., Boyd, H., & Eddy, R. G. (2004). Bovine medicine diseases and husbandry of cattle. 2nd ed. Blackwell Publishing Company, USA.

[2] Arthur, G. H. (2001). *Arthur's Veterinary Reproduction and Obstetrics.*, Eighth Ed., 430-767.

[3] Ball, P. J. H., & Peters, A. R. (2004). Reproduction in Cattle. *Fibiol,* 3, 1-13, 10.1002/9780470751091.

[4] Baxter, S. J., & Ward, W. R. (1997). Incidence of foetal loss in dairy cattle after pregnancy diagnosis using an ultrasound scanner. *Vet Rec.;*, 140, 287-288.

[5] Beal, W. E., Perry, R. C., & Corah, L. R. (1992). The use of ultrasound in monitoring reproductive physiology of beef cattle. *J. Anim. Sci.*, 70, 924-929.

[6] Beal, W. E., Edwards, R. B., & Kearnan, J. M. (1989). Use of B-mode, linear array ultrasonography for evaluating the technique of bovine artificial insemination. *J. Dairy Sci.*, 72, 2198 EOF-202 EOF.

[7] Beghelli, V., Boiti, C., Parmigiani, E., & Barbacini, S. (1986). Pregnancy diagnosis and embryonic mortality in the cow. In: JM Sreenan and MG Diskin (Ed.), *Embryonic Mortality in Farm Animals.*, Martinus Nijhoff, Boston,, 159-167.

[8] Boyd, J. S., & Omran, S. N. (1991). Diagnostic ultrasonography of the bovine female reproductive tract. *In practice*, 13, 109-118.

[9] Boyd, J. S., Omran, S. N., & Ayliffe, T. R. (1988). Use of a high frequency transducer with real time B-mode ultrasound scanning to identify early pregnancy in cows. *Vet. Rec.*, 123, 8-11.

[10] Chaffaux, S., Reddy, G. N. S., Vaton, F., & Thibier, M. (1986). Transrectal real-time ultrasound scanning for diagnosing pregnancy and for monitoring embryonic mortality in dairy cattle. *Anim. Reprod. Sci.,*, 10, 193-200.

[11] Curran, S., Pierson, R. A., & Ginther, O. J. (1986). Ultrasonographic appearance of the bovine conceptus from days 20 through 60. *J. Amer. Vet. Med. Assoc.*, 189, 1295 EOF-302 EOF.

[12] Curran, S. (1986). Bovine foetal development. J Am. Vet Med. Assoc., , 189, 1295-1302.

[13] Diskin, M. G., & Sreenan, J. M. (1980). Fertilization and embryonic mortality rates in beef heifers after artificial insemination. *J. Reprod. Fertil.,*, 59, 463-468.

[14] Driancourt, M. A., Philipon, P., Locatelli, A., Jacques, E., & Webb, R. (1988). Are differences in gonadotrophin concentrations involved in the control of ovulation rate in Romanov and Uede-France ewes? *J. Reprod. Fertil.,*, 83, 509.

[15] Driancourt, M. A., Thatcher, W. W., Terqui, M., & Andrieu, D. (1991). Dynamics of ovarian follicular development in cattle during the oestrous cycle, early pregnancy and in response to PMSG. *Domest. Anim. Endocrinol.,*, 2, 209-21.

[16] Evans, A. C. O. (2003). Characteristics of ovarian follicle development in domestic animals. *Reprod. Domes. Anim.*, 38, 240-246.

[17] Evans, A. C. O., Duffy, P., Hynes, N., & Boland, M. P. (2000). Waves of follicle development during the oestrous cycle in sheep. *Theriogenology,*, 53, 699-715.

[18] Fortune, J. E., Sirois, J., & Quirk, S. M. (1988). The growth and differentiation of ovarian follicles during the bovine oestrous cycle. *Theriogenology,*, 29, 95-109.

[19] Fricke, P. M. (2002). Scanning the future-ultrasonography as a reproductive management tool for dairy cattle. *J. Dairy Sci.*, 85, 1918 EOF-26 EOF.

[20] Galland, J. C., Offenbach, L. A., & Spire, M. F. (1994). Measuring the time needed to confirm foetal age in beef heifers using ultrasonographic examination. *Vet. Med.*, 89, 795-804.

[21] Garcia, A., van der Weijden, G. C., Colenbrander, B., & Bevers, M. M. (1999). Monitoring follicular development in cattle by real-time ultrasonography: a review. *Vet. Rec.,*, 145, 334-40.

[22] Ginther, O. J. (1993). Major and minor follicular waves during the equine oestrus cycle. *J Equine Vet Sci*, 13, 18-25.

[23] Godoi, D. B., Gastal, E. L., & Gastal, M. O. (2002). A comparative study of follicular dynamics between lactating and non-lactating mares: effect of the body condition. *Theriogenology*, 58, 553-556.

[24] Hansar, E., Lemma, A., & Yilma, T. (2011). Confirmation of oestrus observed by dairy owners through gynaecological examination of animals presented for artificial insemination. As part of a DVM thesis, Addis Ababa University, School of Veterinary Medicine.

[25] Jemal, H., Lemma, A., & Yilma, T. (2012). Study on factors affecting the success of artificial insemination program in cattle; Siltie zone. As part of MSc thesis, Faculty of Veterinary Medicine, Addis Ababa University.

[26] Kähn, W. (1992). Ultrasonography as a diagnostic tool in female animal reproduction. *Anim Reprod Sci.,*, 28, 1-10.

[27] Kastelic, J. P., Curran, S., & Ginther, O. J. (1989). Accuracy of ultrasonography for pregnancy diagnosis on days 10 to 22 in heifers. *Theriogenology*, 813 EOF-20 EOF.

[28] Lamb, G. C., Miller, B. L., Traffas, V., & Corah, L. R. (1997). Oestrus detection, first service conception, and embryonic death in beef heifers synchronized with MGA and prostaglandin. *Kansas AES report of progress*, 783, 97.

[29] Lamb, G. C. (2001). Reproductive Real-Time Ultrasound Technology: An Application for improving Calf Crop in Cattle Operations. In:, *Factors Affecting Calf Crop: Biotechnology of Reproduction.*, Ed. M.J. Fields., 231-153.

[30] Lamb, G. C., & Fricke, P. M. (2005). Ultrasound- early pregnancy diagnosis and foetal sexing. *Proceedings, Applied Reproductive Strategies in Beef Cattle,*, Reno, Nevada.

[31] Lemma, A., & Kebede, S. (2011). The effect of mating system and herd size on reproductive performance of dairy cows in market oriented urban dairy farms in and around Addis Ababa. *Revue Méd. Vét.,*, 162, 526-530.

[32] Meyers, P. J. (2002). Early embryonic mortality. *Horse Health care- Reproduction and breeding.*, Meyers Equine Clinic Hillsburgh, Ontario, Canada.

[33] Müller, E., & Wittkowski, G. (1986). Visualization of male and female characteristics of bovine foetuses by real-time ultrasonics. *Theriogenology*, 25, 571.

[34] Noble, K. M., Tebble, J. E., Harvey, D., & Dobson, H. (2000). Ultrasonography and hormone profiles of persistent ovarian follicles (cysts) induced with low doses of progesterone in cattle. *Journal of Reproduction and Fertility*, 120, 361-366.

[35] Palmer, E., & Driancourt, M. A. (1980). Use of ultrasound echography in equine gynaecology. *Theriogenology,*, 13, 203-216.

[36] Perry, T. C. (1991). *Reproduction in domestic animals*, 4th ed., Los Angeles Academic Press. Los Angeles,, 670.

[37] Pierson, R. A., & Ginther, O. J. (1984). Ultrasonography for detection of pregnancy and study of embryonic development in heifers. *Theriogenology*, 225 EOF-33 EOF.

[38] Romano, J. E., & Magee, D. (2001). Applications of trans-rectal ultrasonography in cow/heifer reproduction. In:, *Annual Food Conference proceeding. Conception to Parturition: Fertility in Texas Beef cattle.*, College of Veterinary Medicine. June 2-3. Texas A & M University,, 99-104.

[39] Smith, M. W., & Stevenson, J. S. (1995). Fate of the dominant follicle, embryonal survival, and pregnancy rates in dairy cattle treated with prostaglandin F2α and progestins in the absence or presence of a functional corpus luteum. *J. Anim. Sci.,*, 73, 3743-3751.

[40] Stroud, B. (2006). Bovine Foetal Sexing Using Ultrasound. *Proceedings, Applied Reproductive Strategies in Beef Cattle,*, Stoney Creek Inn, St. Joseph, Missouri, USA.

[41] Szenci, O., Beckers, J. F., Humblot, P., Sulon, J., Sasser, G., Taverne, M. A. M., Varga, J., Baltusen, R., & Shekk, G. (1998). Comparison of ultrasonography, bovine pregnancy-specific protein B, and bovine pregnancy-associated glycoprotein 1 tests for pregnancy detection in dairy cows. *Theriogenology*, 50, 77-88.

[42] Taverne, M. A. M., Szenci, O., Szetag, J., & Piros, A. (1985). Pregnancy diagnosis in cows with linear-array real-time ultrasound scanning: a preliminary note. *Vet. Quarterly*, 7, 264-270.

[43] Vandeplassche, G. M., Wesson, J. A., & Ginther, O. J. (1981). Behavioural, follicular and gonadotropin changes during the oestrus cycle in donkeys. *Theriogenol.,*, 16, 239-249.

[44] Vasconcelos, J. L. M., Silcox, R. W., Lacerda, J. A., Pursley, J. R., & Wiltbank, M. C. (1997). Pregnancy rate, pregnancy loss, and response to heat stress after AI at 2 different times from ovulation in dairy cows. *Biol. Reprod.,*, 56, 140.

[45] Lemma, A., Schwartz, H. J., & Bekana, M. (2006). Application of ultrasonography in the study of the reproductive system of tropical Jennies (species Equus asinus). *Trop. Anim. Health and Prod.*, 38, 267-274.

Chapter 9

Energy Management of Mature Mammalian Spermatozoa

Joan E. Rodríguez-Gil

Additional information is available at the end of the chapter

http://dx.doi.org/10.5772/51711

1. Introduction

The ultimate goal of a mammalian sperm is the transmission of paternal genome to the next generation. To achieve this goal, mammalian spermatozoa are very specialized cells, which have a precise cellular design in dependence on the evolutionary reproductive strategy chosen by each species. This specificity is a very important point, since aspects such as the exact point of ejaculate deposition, oestrous time-lapse, number of males mated with a single female and number and sequence of oocytes released in a single ovulation will be key factors in the modulation of sperm function in order to yield optimal "in vivo" fertility rates. A practical consequence of this specificity is that the functional features that distinguish sperm from one species cannot be extrapoled to other species, hindering thus the assumption of an overall picture to explain mammalian sperm function. Furthermore, the extraordinary complexity of the molecular mechanisms implied in the control and modulation of mammalian mature sperm functions makes impossible to a complete description of these mechanisms in the limited space of this chapter. In this way, this chapter will be devoted to a succinct overview of the mechanisms by which mature mammalian sperm manage their energy levels, with a special emphasis in the observed differences among species and also during their entire life span of sperm from ejaculation. For this purpose, this chapter is centered in the description of specific, very important and punctual aspects of sperm energy metabolism. The first aspect is the type of energy sources, both external and internal, that mammalian sperm can utilize to obtain energy. The second aspect is centered in the main metabolic pathways that mammalian sperm utilize to obtain energy, as well as in the basic control mechanisms that modulate these pathways. The third point will involve the precise role that mitochondria play in the control of the overall mammalian sperm function. Finally, the fourth and last point will be focused in the existence of separate metabolic mammalian sperm phenotypes as the result of the precise evolutionary strategy launched by each species to optimize fertility.

2. Mature mammalian spermatozoon: a dynamic cell with changing energy necessities during its lifetime.

A common characteristic of mature mammalian sperm among species is that these cells are dynamic structures, which must underlie dramatic functional changes during their entire life span, from ejaculation to syngamia. These functional changes, in turn, will imply equally dramatic changes in all aspects of sperm energy management, from external energy sources to energy-consuming functions such as specific motion patterns or capacitation-linked cellular and membrane changes. Thus, a succinct description of the most important changes of mammalian sperm function from ejaculation is needed to a better understanding of the observed changes in sperm energy management during their life span.

Ejaculation implies the launching of a rapid succession of events that completely changes sperm physiology. Thus, ejaculated spermatozoa acquire a fast motion pattern; which is accompanied with several changes in cell membrane composition. The main responsible for these changes are seminal plasma, which contacts with spermatozoa during ejaculation. Composition of seminal plasma is complex. Even worse, seminal plasma has a totally different composition when comparing among different species. An example of this is the monosaccharide composition of seminal plasma. We can detect a wide variety of different sugars, such as glucose, fructose and sorbitol. Moreover, the concentration of these sugars is completely different. Thus, whereas fructose is the main sugar in species like human, glucose is present in significant amount in species like boar [48]. The main monosaccharide present in horse seminal plasma is, at the contrary, sorbitol [42], whereas species like dog has not any monosaccharide in significant concentrations [44, 48]. A similar pattern can be found when analyzing seminal plasma proteins. Thus, whereas dog has practically only one protein, which is characterized by its arginine esterase activity [10], other species such as boar and ram has a wide variety of proteins, including a membrane-protective protein family [8, 56].

What could be the main reason for the enormous differences in composition among seminal plasma from separate species? Investigators can only speculate regarding this point. However, it would be reasonable to suppose that the main reason for these differences is the very specific evolutionary reproductive strategies developed in each species to optimize their fertilizing abilities. In this way, it is logical to suppose that seminal plasma of one long-lived species like dog, would have completely separate characteristics to the seminal plasma of other shorter-lived species, like bull. It is noteworthy that dog spermatozoa have to survive for relatively long periods inside the bitch genital tract and, moreover, must be prepared to compete against spermatozoa from other individuals. On the contrary, bull spermatozoa is adapted to a shorter life-span, since the time lapse between ejaculation and cow ovulation is very short indeed. In any case, seminal plasma has some common features among species intended to solve common problems that spermatozoa find after ejaculation. Thus, seminal plasma must contain components that activate sperm motility. This is absolutely essential in species in which ejaculation is carried out either at the vaginal vestibulum or at cervix. In these placements, the female genital tract presents a very active immunological system, which is further activated during oestrus [23]. This very active system will eliminate all spermatozoa that would not be enough fast or enough fortunate to leave the area and, in this way, sperm motility must be activated immediately after ejaculation. A wide array of seminal plasma components have been identified as motility activators. From these, probably the most known are prostaglandins, which have been found as a common seminal plasma component in several species like human and bovine [25, 52], although there are other components that plays a role as motility activators. Regarding prostaglandins, it has been described that their motility activation role is not mediated by receptors [49]. The activation of this non-receptor pathway would evolve the activation of specific energy-consuming pathways, pointing thus the importance of a fine regulation of the sperm energy metabolism in order to optimize sperm function.

Notwithstanding, seminal plasma must contain other components than those merely acting as motility activators. In this way, functions such as protection against immunological system of female genital tract and signaling to achieve total "in vivo" capacitation into the oviduct are also very important roles associated with seminal plasma. As in case of motility activation, each species will contain separate compounds in their seminal plasma in order to achieve these roles and, at this moment, this is a poorly understood investigation field. Another possible role for seminal plasma is as energy source for the first steps of spermatozoa after ejaculation. Thus, plasma seminal sugars could be a feasible energy source. However, it is difficult to understand why seminal plasma in all species does not contain glucose as their main energy source, since glucose is the most important energy-producing monosaccharide for all of mammalian tissues. Instead of this, seminal plasma contains other sugars, specially fructose, but also sorbitol and other [6, 28, 32, 33, 36, 42, 45], which are not as efficient as glucose as primary energy sources (see as an example in boar sperm [36]. Again, investigators can only speculate on this point. However, recent data from our laboratory seem to indicate that sugars could play a role of specific sperm function modulator besides their energy-fuelling role. This point would be developed in a more in depth manner when discussing external energy sources of sperm, although the possibility that seminal plasma monosaccharides play another role than that of energy sources can be seriously considered.

In any case, after ejaculation only a small percentage of ejaculated spermatozoa are able to leave the ejaculation placement and subsequently they reach oviduct after their uterine transit. Of course, energy requirements of sperm that are in course to the oviduct through uterus are totally different to those immediately after ejaculation. Freshly ejaculated spermatozoa require an energy metabolism in which energy was rapidly generated, in order to support the great amount of energy required by spermatozoa to activate for leaving the ejaculation point. In contrast, spermatozoa that have reached uterus do not require this fast and great energy consumption. In this way, their energy requirements would be much less great and imperative. This is especially important in those species, like pig [31], in which transport through uterus is mainly carried out by uterine peristaltic contractions rather by the sperm motion by itself. This drop in energy requirements will be surely linked to a change in energy-fuelling pathways, although at this moment the changes suffered by energy metabolism during this step are not well known.

However, this is not the last change that mammalian sperm metabolism has to suffer in their life time. Once sperm reach oviduct, they rest in the oviductal crypts until their re-activation, following ovulation. This resting step is of the utmost importance, since at this point sperm, in tightly contact with oviductal cells, reach full capacitated status [14, 55]. Capacitation implies a myriad of functional and structural changes, like loss of cell membrane cholesterol, increase in tyrosine, serine and threonine phosphorylation levels of a wide array of separate proteins and intracellular calcium mobilization, whose full description is not possible in this chapter (see [52, 53] as reviews). Capacitation, however, has a great interest in the sense that its full achievement again implies new energy requirements to carry out processes like the increase in tyrosine phosphorylation of specific sperm proteins, such as pro-acrosin [13, 19]. This new requirements will imply again new changes in energy metabolism, which will be closely linked to the progressive changes that sperm function must suffer during this period.

Finally, remnant sperm will be loaded from the oviductal crypts in order to undergo oocyte penetration. In this period, capacitated sperm adopt a totally specific motility pattern known as hyperactivated motility, with separate characteristics depending on the studied species [51]. Once reached the oocyte, sperm have to penetrate it, launching a series of energy-consuming processes like adherence to oocyte zona pellucida and subsequent acrosome exocytosis [29]. Again, energy requirements will change when comparing with other sperm life–span steps. In this sense, acrosome exocytosis will need a fast and intense energy burst and, in fact, it has been described that progesterone-induced acrosome exocytosis in boar sperm that were previously subjected to "in vitro" capacitation is simultaneous to an intense and transitory increase in O_2 consumption, which would correspond to transitory mitochondria activation [43].

What are the main conclusions that can be yielded? The basic conclusion from all of this information would be that the dramatic changes that undergo mammalian spermatozoa from ejaculation to oocyte penetration must be accompanied by concomitant, dramatic changes in their energy regulating mechanisms. Little is known regarding how mammalian sperm modulate these changes, and this is one of the most challenging investigation fields that is currently open in the study of mammalian sperm function.

3. Energy sources for mammalian spermatozoa

Energy production requires easy availability of energy substrates. In a general sense, any eukaryotic cell can obtain energy from either external or internal sources. External sources can be very different, from monosaccharides to lipids, whereas internal sources are mainly polysaccharides such as glycogen and lipids, although other internal sources can be aminoacids and other. Regarding mammalian sperm, separate external and also internal energy sources have been described, offering thus a view not radically different to that observed in other eukaryotic cells. Notwithstanding, there are several characteristics that differentiates mammalian sperm to other eukaryotic cells in this point. Thus, the sequence of rapid location changes that underwent spermatozoa after ejaculation implies that they are synchronically placed in very separate locations inside female genital tract. This phenomenon will imply separate availability of external energy substrates, depending on the exact placement of spermatozoa. Moreover, the majority of cells integrated in a mammalian body will obtain their external energy sources directly from blood. This is not the case of spermatozoa, which are not keeping in direct contact with blood during their entire life. In this way, external energy sources might came from secretions of cells from the female genital tract or from seminal plasma. This implies that sperm must have very efficient mechanisms to uptake external energy resources, which will not be directly directed towards them. Moreover, and centering on seminal plasma as energy source, the time lapse that ejaculated sperm are in close contact with seminal plasma is, in fact, short. In fact, in species in which the ejaculated volume is short and rapidly placed inside a female genital tract of large size, like cow, contact between sperm and seminal plasma is very short, indeed. In any case, after ejaculation, both sperm and seminal plasma will immediately contact with secretions from the female genital tract. In this manner, sperm would be able to simultaneously find energy sources from both seminal plasma and the female genital tract. Only in species in which the volume of the ejaculate was very voluminous, like porcine, sperm will contact seminal plasma during a significant time lapse. Taking into account all of this information, it seems obvious that the adequate sperm external energy sources intake will depend of two main factors. The first factor will be the efficiency of external energy sources uptake mechanisms that sperm have developed. The second factor will be the specific mixture of external energy sources that sperm find in their journey inside the female genital tract. This mixture will came from both seminal plasma and female genital tract secretions, with predominance from one or the other source depending on the species and the exact location inside the genital tract.

All of this digression has been only centered in the origin of sperm external energy sources. However, what are exactly these energy sources? There is a general consensus in pointing at monosaccharides as the main energy sources for mammalian sperm [46]. Notwithstanding, sperm can utilize other substances than monosaccharides. Thus, boar sperm is able to utilize a wide range of substances, such as glycerol, lactate, pyruvate and citrate [26, 27, 37]. Other species are able to utilize also non-monosaccharide substrates as energy sources, although more information is needed to clarify this point (see as examples [22, 50]). The utilization of non-monosaccharide substrates as energy sources raises the question of the usefulness of these substrates. It has been suggested that these substrates could be an alternative in circumstances in which monosaccharide availability was limited [27, 37]. However, a thorough study of the energy substrates content that is present in each segment of the female genital tract is lacking, even in the best studied species. This impedes the complete elucidation of this suggestion. Despite this, the role of non-monosaccharide substrates as external energy sources for mammalian spermatozoa deserves a more in-depth study in order to clarify its biological importance and role.

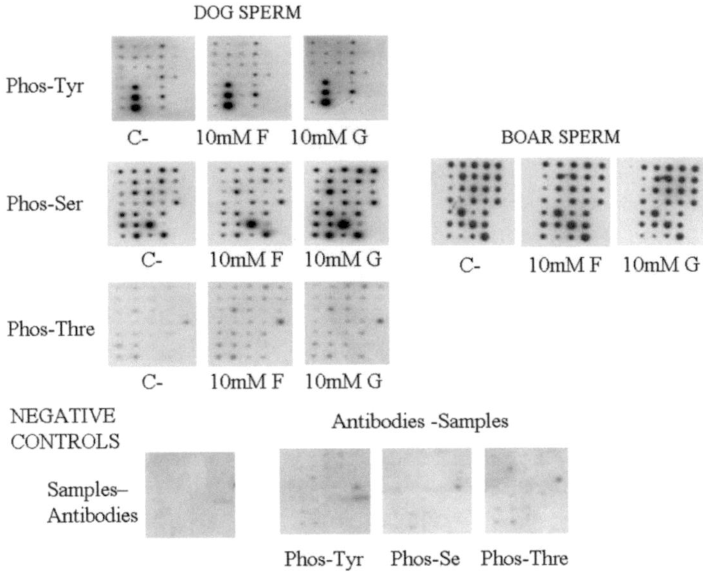

Figure 1. Mini-array analysis of the tyrosine, serine and threonine phosphorylation status of several proteins involved in the regulation of cell cycle and overall cell function in dog and boar spermatozoa after incubation with glucose or fructose. Dog and boar spermatozoa were incubated for 5 min in the absence (C-) or presence of either 10mM fructose (10mM F) or 10mM glucose (10mM G). The tyrosine- (Phos-Tyr), serine- (Phos-Ser) and threonine-phosphorylation (Phos-Thre) levels of each spot in the mini-arrays were then analysed. The figure shows a representative image for five separate experiments. Figure excerpted from [17]).

Turning on monosaccharides, one of the most intriguing questions is the ability of sperm to utilize a variety of sugars that are present, at east in seminal plasma. As indicated above, this is a very difficult question to study, since the sugars composition of seminal plasma is very different among species. In this sense, there are a significant number of species in which fructose is the main sugar, like human or mice [32]. However, in other species, like boar, fructose is not predominant [6, 32]. The main sugar in horse is not fructose or glucose, but sorbitol [42]. This sorbitol is further converted in fructose through the action of the enzyme sorbitol dehydrogenase, despite of old works indicating that horse sperm were not able to metabolize sorbitol [42]. Finally, there are also species, like dog, which lacks any monosaccharide in its seminal plasma [44, 48]. Another intriguing question is the mere presence of sugars, like fructose and sorbitol that are not typical in any other animal tissue. In fact, both fructose and sorbitol are typical vegetal sugars, without any significant presence in animals, excepting in mammalian seminal plasma. It is noteworthy that the utilization of sugars like fructose, sorbitol and mannose by sperm of species like boar and dog of is in fact less effective in order to obtain energy than that of glucose [36, 45]. The greater effectiveness of glucose is mainly linked to a greater sensitivity to the hexokinase system, which phosphorylates sugars as a first step in their metabolization pathway [36, 45]. Taking into account this lower efficiency, it is difficult to understand the biological logics to utilize sugars like fructose or sorbitol as mere energy sources for sperm. Another explanation for this apparent contradiction would be that non-glucose monosaccharides could exert other roles than that of mere energy sources. In this sense, incubation of dog sperm with fructose induced a specific decrease of serine phosphorylation levels of several proteins with key roles in the regulation of sperm cell function, such as protein kinases Akt, PI3 kinase, ERK-1 and protein kinase C ([17] and Figure 1). Strikingly, the incubation with glucose induced a specific increase in the serine phosphorylation levels of other key regulatory proteins, like c-kit, Raf-1, tyrosine kinase and several protein phosphatases ([17] and Figure 1) These effects might induce sugar-specific changes in the overall dog sperm function. On the contrary, the incubation of boar sperm with either glucose or fructose did not induce any of the specific actions observed in dog sperm ([17] and Figure 1). All of these results clearly indicate that sugars can have a sugar- and species-specific action as signaling compounds, modulating thus sperm function in a closely-linked manner, depending on the moment in which sperm and sugar were kept in contact. In this way, the idea of seminal plasma sugars as mere energy sources would be dismissed and being substituted by another idea; sugars as both energy sources and direct sperm function modulators in a simultaneous and coordinated form.

External sources, however, are not the only possibility found by mammalian sperm to obtain energy. Sperm can obtain energy also from endogenous sources. One of the most studied sources is glycogen. The presence of a functional glycogen metabolism has been demonstrated in several species, such as dog, boar, horse, ram and bonnet monkey [5], although no glycogen was found in other species like mice and rat [3]. The primary role of these internal energy sources would be, logically, the maintenance of a limited energy reservoir, although this could not be a universal function. In fact, dog sperm glycogen plays a role in the achievement of "in vitro" capacitation in a medium without glucose by being a key intermediate metabolite in the obtainment of energy through gluconeogenesis, which was essential to the achievement of the capacitated status [1, 2]. Thus, in dog sperm, glycogen plays an important role as capacitation regulator, besides its energy reservoir role. In this manner, a more in-depth sturdy of the exact role of glycogen should be needed to obtain a clearer picture of the utilization of endogenous substrates as energy sources in sperm.

4. Main metabolic pathways to obtain energy and control mechanisms involved in the coordination of energy management of mammalian sperm

If monosaccharides are considered as the most important exogenous energy source for mammalian sperm, the question of the precise metabolic pathways by which mature mammalian sperm obtain energy is relatively straightforward. Thus, the main metabolic pathway is glycolysis. The preeminence of glycolysis in freshly ejaculated sperm has been demonstrated in species like bull, mice and boar [21, 33, 39]. In fact, in species like boar, at least the 95% of the energy obtained from glucose is obtained through the glycolytic pathway in freshly obtained ejaculates [33]. The explanation of the glycolysis preeminence in these species is easy to understand. Glycolysis would reach high velocity rates taking from a very high velocity of sugars intake and phosphorylation. This will be due to the very high sensitivity to sugars of both GLUTs monosaccharide transporters and overall hexokinase activity. In fact, glycolytic rate is so high in species like bull that it rarely achieve the theoretical stoichiometric ATP yield of the glycolytic pathway, living thus to the establishment of an active substrate cycling, important to the maintenance of motility [21]. In fact, the ability of generate energy of a specific sugar would depend on the ability of each sugar to be uptaken and subsequent phosphorylated. In this way, it is important to remind that this sensitivity changes upon a sugar- and species-specific basis. Thus, as described above and taking porcine sperm as a basis, it is important to remind that the velocity by which glucose is phosphorylated and then incorporated to the glycolytic flux is greater than that observed by other sugars like fructose, sorbitol and mannose [36]. The ability of each species to utilize each separate sugar will be then different, depending on the specific machinery that sperm have in order to uptake and further phosphorylate monosaccharides. In fact, this machinery can be more different among species than that previously thought. As an example, dog sperm have two separate hexokinase activities. The first has a very high sensitivity for sugars as glucose, with a Km of about 0.1 mM. The second hexokinase activity has much lover glucose sensitivity, with kinetic properties very similar to those described for hepatic glucokinase [16]. This sophisticated machinery makes dog sperm able to develop a dual reactivity to react against very separate glucose concentrations, specifically changing sperm function in contact with environments with these separate characteristics. Remarkably, sperm from other species such as boar have not any glucokinase-like activity [16], reflecting thus a species-specific reactivity against glucose that is inititated at the very start of the glucose utilization pathway.

The final sugar utilization step is the entry of pyruvate obtained at the end of glycolysis into mitochondria to be subsequent degraded into the mitochondrial respiration system. There is not a universal agreement regarding the importance of mitochondria-based energy obtainment. In this way, an optimal mitochondrial function has been related not only with sperm motility in bull [18], horse [20], ram [34] and mouse [39] but also with fertilization ability in human (30). However, gene knock-out of the glycolytic enzyme glyceraldehyde-phosphate dehydrogenase (GAPDH) in transgenic mice caused the appearance of non-motile sperm and a significant reduction of the ATP content (10% of the total) despite having no deficiency in oxygen consumption [38]. This seems to imply that although a correct mitochondrial function is needed to the maintenance of an optimal sperm function, mitochondrial respiration would not be the most important role of mitochondria to exert their activity. Another explanation would be that mitochondrial respiration would not be important in the maintenance of the overall energy status of sperm, although it would be of the utmost importance in the maintenance of punctual aspects of sperm function. In this sense, progesterone-induced acrosome exocytosis of boar sperm subjected to a previous "in vitro" capacitation is concomitant with a rapid, intense and transitory burst of oxygen consumption [42]. Moreover, unpublished results from our laboratory show that the inhibition of this oxygen consumption burst is concomitant with an almost complete lack of progesterone-induced acrosome exocytosis (Figure 2 and data not shown). These results are concomitant with overall low levels of oxygen consumption, which in fact indicate that the majority of ATPs obtained by boar sperm do not come from mitochondrial respiration [33]. However, the results seem to indicate that the minority mitochondrial respiration is essential to obtain a feasible progesterone-induced acrosome exocytosis.

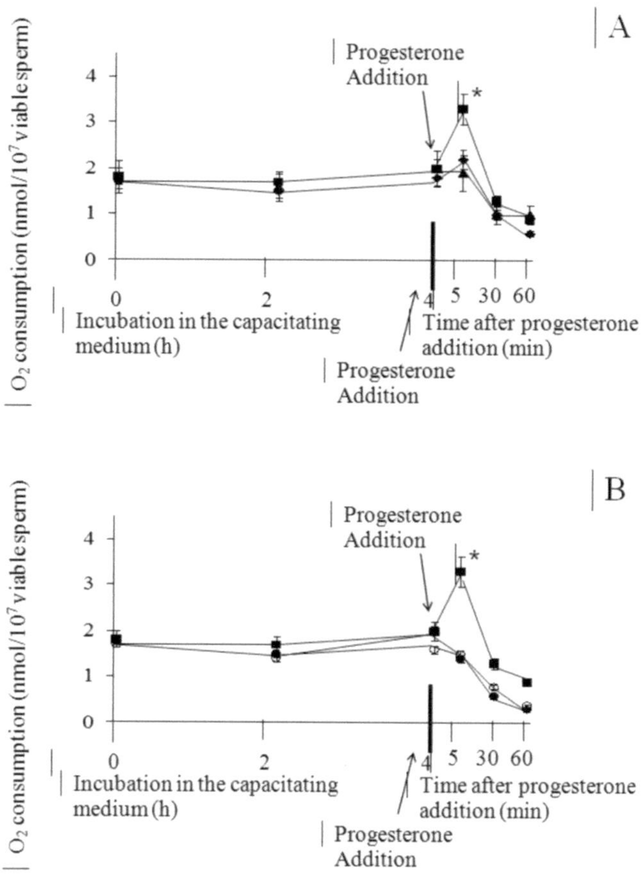

Figure 2. Rhythm of O_2 consumption of boar sperm subjected to "in vitro" capacitation and subsequent "in vitro" acrosome reaction in the presence or absence of olygomycin A or in Ca^{2+}-depleted capacitation medium. Boar sperm were incubated for 4h and then were added with 10 µg/mL progesterone and subjected to a further incubation for 60 min. A): Sperm cells incubated in a standard capacitation medium or in media added with 2.4 µM olygomycin A. ■: Control cells. ◆: Spermatozoa incubated in capacitation medium added with 2.4 µM olygomycin A from the beginning of the incubation. ▲: Spermatozoa incubated in a standard capacitation medium for 4h and subsequent added with 10 µg/mL progesterone and 2.4 µM olygomycin A together. B): Sperm cells incubated in a standard capacitation medium or in Ca^{2+}-depleted media. ○: Spermatozoa incubated in capacitation medium without Ca^{2+} and added with 2 mM EGTA from the beginning of the experiments. ●: Spermatozoa incubated in a standard capacitation medium for 4h and subsequent added with 10 µg/mL progesterone and 2 mM EGTA together Results are expressed as means ±S.E.M. for 7 separate experiments. Asterisks indicate significant ($P<0.05$) differences when compared with the respective Control values. Results excerpted from [43]) and unpublished data from our laboratory.

However, as exposed above, monosaccharides are not the only energy source that sperm can utilize. Other substrates, such as citrate and lactate, can be utilized to obtain energy, at least in several mammalian species. The ways by which mammalian sperm utilize these non-monosaccharide substrates have not been as thoroughly studied as those linked to monosaccharide metabolization. In this way, boar sperm have been one of the most studied species. In this species, extracellular citrate and lactate are utilized after their intake by metabolization through the Krebs cycle [37]. This metabolization is the same than that detailed for many other cellular types. However, sperm utilization of citrate and lactate has several specific features. Thus, a sperm-specific lactate dehydrogenase (LDH) isozyme has been described in several species [12, 27, 37, 40, 41]. This specific isozyme, named LDH-X is the most important LDH form in sperm in which it has been described, such as boar [27], whereas its activity presents several differentiate features. In this sense, the LDH-X is distributed in both soluble and non-soluble fractions of sperm extracts obtained through sonication [37], indicating thus the existence of a specific distribution pattern of this LDH-X in sperm. Moreover, the kinetic characteristics of the LDH are different, depending on the location of the enzyme, either in the soluble or the non-soluble sperm extract fraction [37]. In fact, immunocytochemistry of boar sperm has shown that the LDH-X is mainly located at the midpiece and principal area of the tail, linking thus its activity to the neighboring of mitochondria-located Krebs cycle activity [37]. All of these information clearly indicate that the regulation of sperm LDH activity, and hence lactate metabolism, is regulated in a very complex manner, with mechanisms depending on factors such as the precise location of the key regulatory enzymes. Another interesting feature of both sperm lactate and citrate metabolism is that lactate enters the Krebs cycle through a direct pathway, which does not need its previous conversion to pyruvate [27, 37]. This direct pathway is important, since it not only produces energy, but also relevant levels of reductive potential, allowing sperm to regenerate significant amounts of NAD^+. Regarding citrate, sperm can metabolize it through two simultaneous pathways. The first pathway is through direct utilization by Krebs cycle, yielding CO_2 and ATP. The second pathway is indirect, by following two sequential steps. A first step in which citrate enters into the Krebs cycle. In the second step the metabolites derived from citrate after its pass through the Krebs cycle are directed to the pyruvate carboxylase step, which converted these metabolites in lactate, which, in turn, will be sent to the extracellular medium and again re-entered into the Krebs cycle through the LDH-X step. At first glance, the biological meaning of this second, convoluted pathway is not immediately understood. However, if the maintenance of a correct NAD^+/NADH equilibrium is considered as basic to maintain a proper sperm function, the main objective of this second, indirect pathway would be not the obtainment of energy, but of reductive potential. In this way, citrate and lactate can have a paramount role not as energy producers, but as reductive potential metabolites.

5. Roles of mitochondria in the control of the overall mature boar sperm function

As previously indicated, the main energy source for mature mammalian sperm are ATPs obtained either through the glycolytic pathway or mitochondrial oxidative pathways. The precise equilibrium between both energy-obtaining pathways will be different among species and in cases like boar and mice, this equilibrium is greatly unbalanced towards glycolysis, which is the overly majoritary energy-obtaining pathway in the presence of sugars like glucose [33, 39)]. This pre-eminence of glycolysis in species like boar and mouse arises to an important question, if sperm mitochondria seem no have a predominant role in these species in obtaining energy, what are their main role? Investigators can only speculate on this point, although there are several data regqarding mainly boar sperm that can aid to obtain a better vision of this issue. The first data correspond to the observation of boar sperm mitochondria ultra-structure (Figure 3). Electron microscope images of boar sperm mitochondria show an organella with very few prominent inner membrane crests. Instead of this, the inner mitochondrial space is mainly occupied by thin and short crests and with an amorphous and homogeneous matrix. This is very different to the classical image for mitochondria, which, like those form hepatocytes, show an inner structure crowded with prominent inner crests. Taking into account that the most important steps of the electronic transport system and subsequent ATP synthesis are structurally linked to inner mitochondrial crests, it is easy to assume that boar sperm mitochondria would be not be very efficient as energy suppliers. In fact, the oxygen consumption rate of boar sperm, which is a direct measure of mitochondrial ability to generate energy, is about 2 magnitude orders lower than that measured in pig hepatocytes [4, 43]. However, this does not preclude that mitochondria-originated energy would not be important for sperm function in species in which glycolysis is the most important energy-synthesizing pathway. Regarding this point, our laboratory has shown that the achievement of a feasible, progesterone-induced "in vitro" acrosome reaction is concomitant with a sudden and intense peak of O_2 consumption rate and also of intracellular ATP levels ([43] and Figures 2,4). Furthermore, unpublished data from our laboratory clearly shows that this peak is not present in conditions in which progesterone-induced acrosome reaction is prevented. These results strongly suggest the existence of a close relationship between mitochondria-generated energy and the achievement of the acrosome reaction, despite of the low energy-efficiency of these organelles.

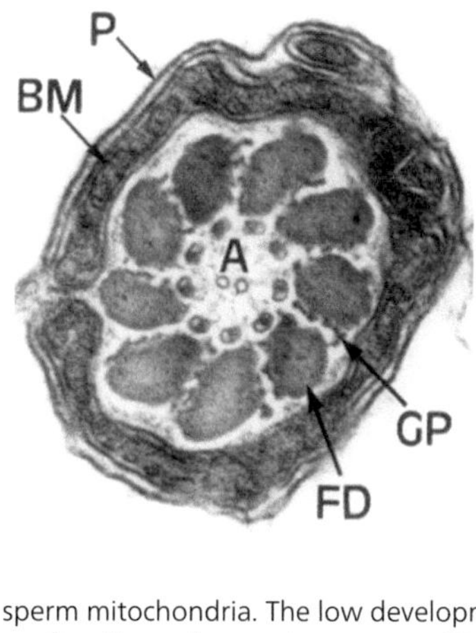

Figure 3. Ultrastructural image of boar sperm mitochondria. The low development of inner crests is noticeable (asterisks). BM: inner mitochondrial membrane. P: cell membrane. A: axoneme. FD: dense fibres. GP: peripheral granules. From [7]).

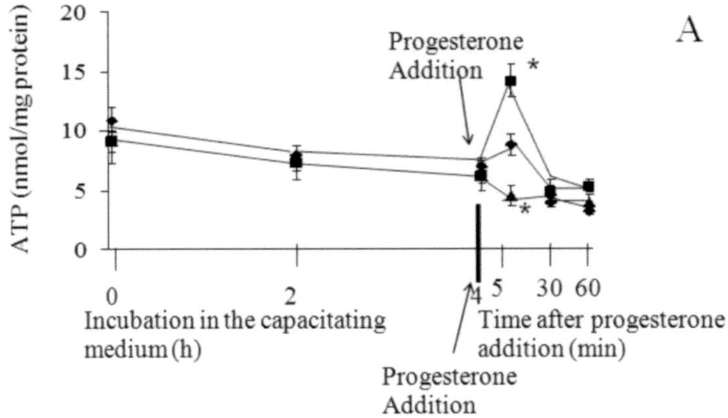

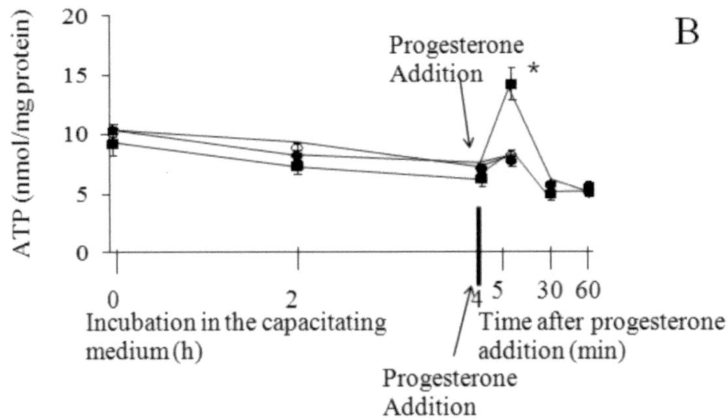

Figure 4. Intracellular ATP levels of boar sperm subjected to "in vitro" capacitation and subsequent "in vitro" acrosome reaction in the presence or absence of olygomycin A or in Ca^{2+}-depleted capacitation medium. Boar sperm were incubated for 4h and then were added with 10 µg/mL progesterone and subjected to a further incubation for 60 min. A): Sperm cells incubated in a standard capacitation medium or in media added with 2.4 µM olygomycin A. ■: Control cells. ◆: Spermatozoa incubated in capacitation medium added with 2.4 µM olygomycin A from the beginning of the incubation. ▲: Spermatozoa incubated in a standard capacitation medium for 4h and subsequent added with 10 µg/mL progesterone and 2.4 µM olygomycin A together. B): Sperm cells incubated in a standard capacitation medium or in Ca^{2+}-depleted media. ○: Spermatozoa incubated in capacitation medium without Ca^{2+} and added with 2 mM EGTA from the beginning of the experiments. ●: Spermatozoa incubated in a standard capacitation medium for 4h and subsequent added with 10 µg/mL progesterone and 2 mM EGTA together Results are expressed as means±S.E.M. for 7 separate experiments. Asterisks indicate significant ($P<0.05$) differences when compared with the respective Control values. Results excerpted from unpublished data from our laboratory.

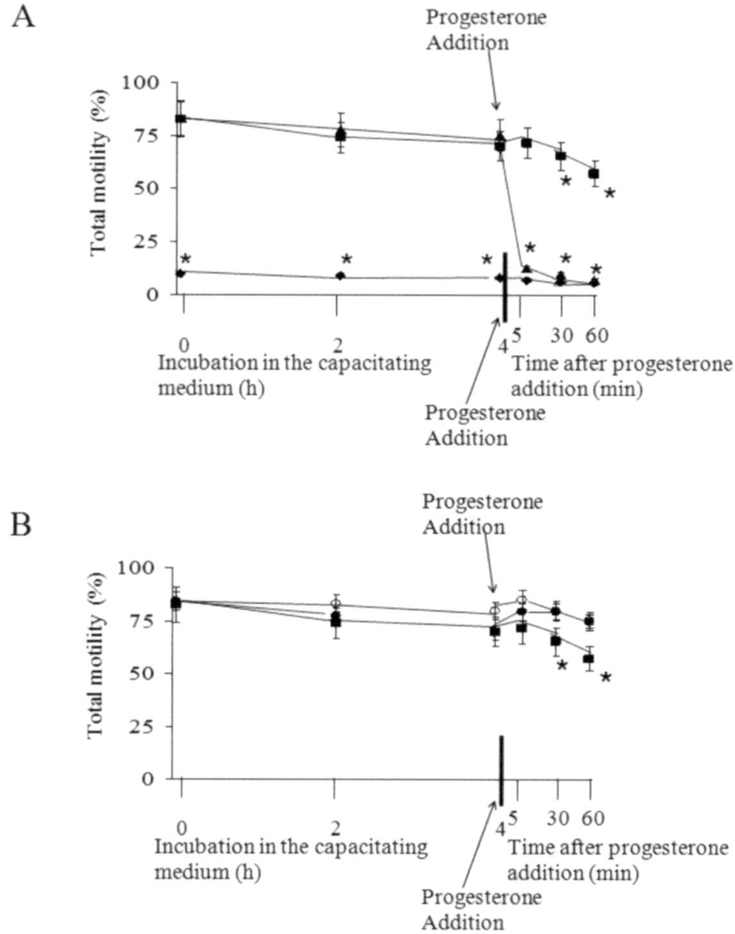

Figure 5. Percentages of total motility of boar sperm subjected to "in vitro" capacitation and subsequent "in vitro" acrosome reaction in the presence or absence of olygomycin A or in Ca^{2+}-depleted capacitation medium. Boar sperm were incubated for 4h and then were added with 10 μg/mL progesterone and subjected to a further incubation for 60 min. Total motility has been defined as the percentage of spermatozoa with a curvilinear velocity (VCL) higher than 20 μm/sec. A): Sperm cells incubated in a standard capacitation medium or in media added with 2.4 μM olygomycin A. ■: Control cells. ◆: Spermatozoa incubated in capacitation medium added with 2.4 μM olygomycin A from the beginning of the incubation. ▲: Spermatozoa incubated in a standard capacitation medium for 4h and subsequent added with 10 μg/mL progesterone and 2.4 μM olygomycin A together. B): Sperm cells incubated in a standard capacitation medium or in Ca^{2+}-depleted media. ○: Spermatozoa incubated in capacitation medium without Ca^{2+} and added with 2 mM EGTA from the beginning of the experiments. ●: Spermatozoa incubated in a standard capacitation medium for 4h and subsequent added with 10 μg/mL progesterone and 2 mM EGTA together Results are expressed as means±S.E.M. for 7 separate experiments. Asterisks indicate significant ($P<0.05$) differences when compared with the respective Control values. Results excerpted from 42) and unpublished data from our laboratory

However, the fact that Krebs cycle seems to be important only in punctual moments of the boar sperm life-time does not necessarily indicate that boar sperm mitochondria are only important in this point. It is noteworthy that mitochondria have much more roles than purely being a mere energy-producing factory. Mitochondria also play a key role in the control of other very important aspects of eukaryotic cells function, like modulation of apoptosis and the control of calcium metabolism. Thus, it is very probable that mitochondria from sperm of species like boar or mouse exert their most important functions on other cellular functional points than energy management. Unpublished results from our laboratory are strongly pointing out this supposition. Thus, the incubation of boar sperm in a capacitation medium in the presence of olygomycin A, a specific inhibitor of the electronic chain and the chemiosmosis steps [11], immobilizes boar sperm and prevent them to achieve "in vitro" capacitation. However, this effect was accomplished without any significant changes in the rhythm of O_2 production and the intracellular ATP levels (Figures 2, 4, 5 and data not shown from our labvoratory). In contrast, the incubation of boar sperm in a capacitation medium without calcium induces an increase in the velocity parameters of these cells, although the achievement of capacitation is also prevented (data not shown). The effect linked to the lack of extracellular calcium however, is again concomitant with no changes in both the rhythm of O_2 production and the intracellular ATP levels (Figures 2, 4 and data not shown). The conclusion from these results is that boar (and probably mice) sperm mitochondria play an important regulatory role in the control of functional aspects such as motility patterns and the achievement of "in vitro" capacitation by ways that are not directly linked to energy production. This opens a new perspective in the manner in which investigators would have to approximate to the understanding of the mitochondria role in the control of sperm function. However, much more work is needed in order to achieve a complete view of this complex phenomenon.

6. Metabolic phenotypes: a result of the separate evolutionary strategies developed by mammals to optimize reproductive indexes

All of data showed above highlight a phenomenon that has not been much explained, although it is well known by all of investigators in this field. This phenomenon is the strong species-specificity that energy obtainment mechanisms show when comparing separate mammals. Differences are so intense that several metabolic phenotypes can be defined, depending on the metabolic characteristics showed by each species. In this manner, there are at least two separate metabolic phenotypes regarding mammalian spermatozoa. The first phenotype will be composed by species in which energy substrates, mainly monosaccharides, will be directed to the practically immediate utilization of all of the assimilated sugars through the appropriate catabolic pathways, especially glycolysis. This specific metabolic phenotype is very common in mammalian sperm, especially in those species, which do not require a long, sperm-survival time-lapse inside the female genital tract such as pig and bull [24, 47]. However, a second phenotype is evident in species where sperm survival inside the female genital tract must be relatively long, such as the dog [15]. In these species, an energy strategy based upon an entirely catabolic metabolism would not be efficient. The optimization of energy Management in relatively long-living sperm like dog would be optimized with the presence of alternative anabolic pathways, such as glycogen synthesis, which allows for the maintenance of a significant mid-to-long intracellular energy reserve. This reserve would play an important role in the maintenance of "in vivo" sperm survival. In fact, as discussed above, the existence of a fully functional glycogen metabolism has been demonstrated in sperm from species like dog, boar, horse and ram [5]. Remarkably, dog sperm shows the most active glycogen metabolism of all of the studied species, in this way accumulating the maximal recorded intracellular levels [5]. As described above, this glycogen plays an important role in the achievement of feasible "in vitro" capacitation [1, 2], reinforcing thus the importance of this anabolic pathway in dog. The importance of glycogen synthesis in dog would be surely linked to another important feature, also described above. It is worth noting that dog sperm is the only studied species so far that shows the presence of two separate hexokinase activities. The first of them is similar to hexokinase-I, which is present in all of the studied mammalian sperm. The second, however, is similar in kinetic and immunologic properties to the hepatic and pancreatic isoform glucokinase [16]. The presence of a glucokinase-like activity in dog sperm but not in other species like boar acquires utmost importance when the precise role that hepatic and pancreatic glucokinase plays is studied. Thus, it is well known that hepatic glucokinase acts as a "metabolistate" that diverts hexoses metabolism to either anabolic or catabolic pathways, depending on factors such as the precise physiologic cell status and sugar extracellular levels [9]. If a similar role for the dog sperm glucokinase-like activity is assumed, the inference that this protein also regulates the entry of energy metabolites in either anabolic or catabolic pathways can be also yielded. These assumptions, notwithstanding will depend on both the precise energy necessities and the extracellular concentrations of sugars inside the female genital tract. Moreover, this "metabolistate" seems to be in the basis of above described, observed differential effects of fructose and glucose in the serine phosphorylation levels of dog sperm proteins like protein kinase C [17]. Thus, dog sperm reaches an even more fine regulation of not only their intracellular energy levels, but also their overall functional status. This very fine regulation would surely increase survival ability of these cells.

These two separate metabolic phenotypes would not surely be the only present among mammalian species. Much more work is needed in order to describe and analyze this phenomenon. In any case, the existence of these metabolic phenotypes would be of the greatest importance. These phenotypes, in fact, will be the reflection of the sperm specialization due to the adoption of separate reproductive strategies among mammals. Thus, these separate evolutive, reproductive strategies will cause the existence of great differences among sperm of separate species not only under a morphological, but also under a metabolic point of view. These differences among species would be, in turn, at the basis of the described differences in vital aspects of sperm function, such as motility patterns and capacitation mechanisms. Finally, these physiological differences would also be reflected in changes in the specific strategy developed to store a particular semen sample from a precise species in optimal conditions.

7. Modulation of energy metabolism as a tool to improve IA results

It seems obvious that a good regulation of the energy regulation mechanisms would be of the utmost importance in order to optimize sperm storage and, hence AI results. Surprisingly, very few investigations have been conducted on this specific point. This could be due to the historical misinterpretation of sperm energy regulatory mechanisms. Historically, these mechanisms has be considered as being simple and linear and, hence of little practical importance [32]. In this way, the majority of semen extenders contain inordinate concentrations of various sugars, like glucose and fructose. The basis for this addition is the thinking that sperm will utilize separate sugars in a similar manner and by linear, concentration-dependent mechanisms. This strategy has at least three weak points. The first point is the fact that the optimal utilization of sugars by sperm is reached to determined concentrations of this sugars. For instance, the optimal utilization rate of glucose by sperm from dog and boar is reached to very low concentrations of the sugar, at about 0.1 mM [16, 36, 37, 45]. This indicates that the addition of low concentrations of sugar to the extenders would be enough to maintain sperm energy levels. This is not followed by the majority of extenders, in which sugars are added to concentrations above 50 mM. At these concentrations, the sperm energy machinery is overrated and non-optimal, despite the fact that cells are stored to low temperatures. The second weak point is the fact that, as described above, sugars could have other effects that being mere energy supplies (see [17]). In this case, the election of either glucose or fructose in a species can influence their ability of survival by modifying specific aspects of sperm functionality. The third weak point is that mammalian sperm are abler to utilize nonglucidic substrates as energy sources. Nonglucidic substrates like lactate and citrate are frequently added to semen extenders in order to play roles that are not related to the maintenance of sperm energy levels. Some of these roles are, for instance, maintenance of osmolarity and pH. However, sperm cells can consume these substances and, in this way, the extender design would lose its conservative properties, since some protective functions (maintenance of osmolarity, pH, etc.) could be impaired when these substances are metabolized by sperm. Following this rationale, the exact proportion of glucose and nonglucidic substrates like citrate and lactate greatly affects several parameters of boar-semen quality analysis during storage at 15ºC-17ºC. Some of the parameters affected by the exact sugar/non-sugar composition of extenders were the membrane integrity, the response to functional tests like the osmotic resistance test and the overall mid-term survival at 15ºC-17ºC [35]. These results strongly suggest that the exact proportion of these substrates, more than their final concentration, is of the greatest importance to optimize the maintenance of sperm function during sperm storage in refrigerated conditions.

As a conclusion, the lack of a proper knowledge of the mechanisms linked to the control of mammalian sperm energy management is hampered a further optimization of the semen extenders utilized in the different species. This would have a detrimental effect in the subsequent AI results obtained with semen stored in sub-optimally designed extenders. This highlights the great interest in more investigations in order to elucidate the exact mechanisms of energy management in all of the domestic mammalian species.

8. Conclusion

Energy management of mature mammalian spermatozoa is a much complex question than that usually devised. This complexity is due to a combination of factors, such as the existence of rapid and profound environmental changes during the entire life of sperm post-ejaculation, as well as the development of many different evolutionary reproductive strategies among mammalian species, which lead sperm to develop specific energetic strategies. In this sense, factors like the time that sperm have to spend inside the female genital tract or the existence of competence among sperm from separate males inside the female will play important roles in the design of an optimal energy management strategy in each mammalian species.

Author details

Joan E. Rodríguez-Gil[1*]

Address all correspondence to: juanenrique.rodriguez@uab.cat

1 Dept. Animal Medicine & Surgery, Autonomous University of Barcelona, Spain

References

[1] Albarracín, J. L., Mogas, T., Palomo, Peña. A., Rigau, T., & Rodríguez-Gil, J. E. (2004a). In vitro" capacitation and acrosome reaction of dog spermatozoa can be feasibly attained in a defined medium without glucose. *Reprod Domest Anim*, 39, 1-7.

[2] Albarracín, J. L., Fernández-Novell, J. M., Ballester, J., Rauch, M. C., Quintero-Moreno, A., Peña, A., Mogas, T., Rigau, T., Yañez, A., Guinovart, J. J., Slebe, J. C., Concha, I. I., & Rodríguez-Gil, J. E. (2004b). Gluconeogenesis-linked glycogen metabolism is important in the achievement of in vitro capacitation of dog spermatozoa in a medium without glucose. *Biol Reprod*, 71, 1437-1445.

[3] Anderson, W. A., & Personne, P. (1970). The localization of glycogen in the spermatozoa of various invertebrate and vertebrate species. *J Cell Biol*, 44, 29-51.

[4] Balis, U. J., Behnia, K., Dwarakanath, B., & Bhatia, S. N. (1999). Oxygen consumption characteristics of porcine hepatocytes. *Metab Eng*, 1, 49-62.

[5] Ballester, J., Fernández-Novell, J. M., Rutllant, J., García-Rocha, M., Palomo, MJ, Mogas, T., Peña, A., Rigau, T., Guinovart, J. J., & Rodríguez-Gil, J. E. (2000). Evidence for a functional glycogen metabolism in mature mammalian spermatozoa. *Mol Reprod Develop*, 56, 207-219.

[6] Baronos, S. (1971). Seminal carbohydrate in boar and stallion. *J Reprod Fertil*, 24, 303-305.

[7] Bonet, S., Briz, M., Pinart, E., Sancho, S., García-Gil, N., & Badia, E. (2000). Morphology of boar spermatozoa. *Bonet S, Durfort M, Egozcu J, eds. Insititu d'Estudis Catalans, Barcelona (Spain)*, 8-47283-533-2.

[8] Calvete, J. J., & Sanz, L. (2007). Insights into structure-function correlations of ungulate seminal plasma proteins. Soc Reprod Fertil Suppl. , 65, 201-215.

[9] Cárdenas, M. L., Cornish-Bowden, A., & Ureta, T. (1998). Evolution and regulatory role of the hexokinases. *Biochim Biophys Acta*, 1401, 242-264.

[10] Chapdelaine, P., Dubé, J. Y., Frenette, G., & Tremblay, R. R. (1984). Identification of arginine esterase as the major androgen-dependent protein secreted by dog prostate and preliminary molecular characterization in seminal plasma. *J Androl*, 5, 206-210.

[11] Chappell, J. B., & Greville, G. D. (1961). Effects of oligomycin on respiration and swelling of isolated liver mitochondria. *Nature*, 190, 502-504.

[12] Coronel, C. E., Burgos, C., Pérez de, Burgos. N. M., Rovai, L. E., & Blanco, A. (1983). Catalytic properties of the sperm-specific lactate dehydrogenase (LDH X or C4) from different species. *J Exp Zool*, 225, 379-385.

[13] Dubé, C., Leclerc, P., Baba, T., Reyes-Moreno, C., & Bailey, J. L. (2005). The proacrosin binding protein, sp32, is tyrosine phosphorylated during capacitation of pig sperm. *J Androl*, 26, 519-28.

[14] Fazeli, A., Duncan, A. E., Watson, P. F., & Holt, W. V. (1999). Sperm-oviduct interaction: induction of capacitation and preferential binding of uncapacitated spermatozoa to oviductal epithelial cells in porcine species. *Biol Reprod*, 60, 879-886.

[15] Feldman, E. C., & Nelson, R. W. (1987). Fertilization. *In: Canine and feline endocrinology and reproduction. Pedersen E, ed.*, 420-421, WB Saunders Co., Philadelphia (USA).

[16] Fernández-Novell, J. M., Ballester, J., Medrano, A., Otaegui, P. J., Rigau, T., Guinovart, J. J., & Rodríguez-Gil, J. E. (2004). The presence of a high-Km hexokinase activity in dog, but not in boar, sperm. *FEBS Lett*, 570, 211-6.

[17] Fernández-Novell, J. M., Ballester, J., Altirriba, J., Ramió-Lluch, L., Barberà, A., Gomis, R., Guinovart, J. J., & Rodríguez-Gil, J. E. (2011). Glucose and fructose as functional modulators of overall dog, but not boar sperm function. *Reprod Fertil Develop*, 23, 468-480.

[18] Garner, D. L., & Thomas, C. A. (1999). Organelle-specific probe JC-1 identifies membrane potential differences in the mitochondrial function of bovine sperm. *Mol Reprod Dev*, 53, 222-229.

[19] Grasa, P., Colás, C., Gallego, M., Monteagudo, L., Muiño-Blanco, T., & Cebrián-Pérez, J. A. (2009). Changes in content and localization of proteins phosphorylated at ty-

rosine, serine and threonine residues during ram sperm capacitation and acrosome reaction. *Reproduction*, 137, 655-667.

[20] Gravance, C. G., Garner, D. L., Baumber, J., & Ball, B. A. (2000). Assessment of equine sperm mitochondrial function using JC-1. *Theriogenology*, 53, 1691-1703.

[21] Hammersted, R. H., & Lardy, H. A. (1983). The effects of substrate cycling on the ATP yield of sperm glycolysis. *J Biol Chem*, 258, 8759-8768.

[22] Hereng, T. H., Elgstøen, K. B. P., Cederkvist, F. H., Eide, L., Jahnsen, T., Skålhegg, BS, & Rosendal., K. R. (2011). Exogenous pyruvate accelerates glycolysis and promotes capacitation in human spermatozoa. *Hum Reprod*, 26, 3249-3263.

[23] Horne, A. W., Stock, S. J., & King, A. E. (2008). Innate immunity and disorders of the female reproductive tract. *Reproduction*, 135, 739-749.

[24] Hunter, R. H. F. (1982). Interrelationships between spermatozoa, the female reproductive tract and the eggs investments. *In: Control of pig reproduction. Cole DJA, Foxcroft GR, eds.*, 49-64, Butterworth Scientific, London.

[25] Jaeger, J. R., & Delcurto, T. (2012). Endogenous prostaglandin F(2α) concentrations in bovine whole semen, seminal plasma, and extended semen. *Theriogenology*, 15, 369-75.

[26] Jones, A. R., Chantrill, L. A., & Cokinakis, A. (1992). Metabolism of glycerol by mature boar spermatozoa. *J Reprod Fertil*, 94, 129-134.

[27] Jones, A. R. (1997). Metabolism of lactate by mature boar spermatozoa. *Reprod Fertil Develop*, 9, 227-232.

[28] Jones, A. R., & Connor, D. E. (2000). Fructose metabolism by mature boar spermatozoa. *J Reprod Fertil*, 94, 129-134.

[29] Kaji, K., & Kudo, A. (2004). The mechanism of sperm-oocyte fusion in mammals. *Reproduction*, 127, 423-429.

[30] Kasai, T., Ogawa, K., Mizuno, K., Nagai, S., Uchida, Y., Ohta, S., Fujie, M., Suzuki, K., Hirata, S., & Hoshi, K. (2002). Relationship between sperm mitochondrial membrane potential, sperm motility, and fertility potential. *Asian J Androl*, 4, 97-110.

[31] Langendijk, P., Soede, N. M., & Kemp, B. (2005). Uterine activity, sperm transport, and the role of boar stimuli around insemination in sows. *Theriogenology*.

[32] Mann, T. (1975). Biochemistry of semen. *In: Handbook of Physiology. Greep RO, Astwood EB, eds.*, 321-347, American Physiology Society, Washington, DC (USA).

[33] Marín, S., Chiang, K., Bassilian, S., Lee-N, W., Boros, P., Fernández-Novell, L. G., Centelles, J. M., Medrano, J. J., Rodríguez-Gil, A., & Cascante, J. E. M. (2003). Metabolic strategy of boar spermatozoa revealed by a metabolomic characterization. *FEBS Lett*, 554, 342-346.

[34] Martínez-Pastor, F., Johannisson, A., Gil, J., Kaabi, M., Anel, L., Paz, P., & Rodríguez-Martínez, H. (2004). Use of chromatin stability assay, mitochondrial stain JC-1, and fluorometric assessment of plasma membrane to evaluate frozen-thawed ram semen. *Anim Reprod Sci*, 84, 121-133.

[35] Medrano, A., Peña, A., Rigau, T., & Rodríguez-Gil, J. E. (2005). Variations in the proportion of glycolytic/non-glycolytic energy substrates modulate sperm membrane integrity and function in diluted boar samples stored at 15-17ºC. *Reprod Domest Anim*, 40, 448-453.

[36] Medrano, A., García-Gil, N., Ramió, L., Rivera, M. M., Fernández-Novell, J. M., Ramírez, A., Peña, A., Briz, M. D., Pinart, E., Concha, I. I., Bonet, S., Rigau, T., & Rodríguez-Gil, J. E. (2006a). Hexose specificity of hexokinase and ADP-dependence of pyruvate kinase play important roles in the control of monosaccharide utilization in freshly diluted boar spermatozoa. *Mol Reprod Dev*, 73, 1179-1199.

[37] Medrano, A., Fernández-Novell, J. M., Ramió, L., Alvarez, J., Goldberg, E., Rivera, M., Guinovart, J. J., Rigau, T., & Rodríguez-Gil, J. E. (2006b). Utilization of citrate and lactate through a lactate dehydrogenase and ATP-regulated pathway in boar spermatozoa. *Mol Reprod Develop*, 73, 369-378.

[38] Miki, K., Qu, W., Goulding, E. H., Willis, W. D., Bunch, D. O., Strader, L. F., Perreault, S. D., Eddy, E. M., & O'Brien, D. A. (2004). Glyceraldehyde 3-phosphate dehydrogenase-S, a sperm-specific glycolytic enzyme, is required for sperm motility and male fertility. *Proc Natl Acad Sci USA*, 101, 16501-16506.

[39] Mukai, C., & Okuno, M. (2004). Glycolysis plays a major role for adenosinetriphosphate supplementation in mouse sperm flagellar movement. *Biol Reprod*, 71, 540-547.

[40] Pan, Y. C., Sharief, F. S., Okabe, M., Huang, S., & Li, S. S. (1983). Amino acid sequence studies on lactate dehydrogenase C4 isozymes from Mouse and rat testes. *J Biol Chem*, 258, 7005-7016.

[41] Pawlowski, R., & Brinkmann, B. (1992). Evaluation of sperm specific lactate dehydrogenase isoenzyme C4 (LDH C4): Application to semen detection in stains. *Int J Legal Med*, 105, 123-126.

[42] Polakoski, K. L., & Kopta, M. (1982). Seminal plasma. In: Biochemistry of mammalian reproduction. Zaneveld, L.J.D. and Chatterton, R.T., eds.,. John Wiley & Sons, New York, 89-117.

[43] Ramió-Lluch, L., Fernández-Novell, J. M., Peña, A., Colás, C., Cebrián-Pérez, J. A., Muiño-Blanco, T., Ramírez, A., Concha, I. I., Rigau, T., & Rodríguez-Gil, J. E. (2011). In vitro" capacitation and acrosome reaction are concomitant with specific changes in mitochondrial activity in boar sperm: evidence for a nucleated mitochondrial activation and for the existence of a capacitation-sensitive subpopulational structure. *Reprod Domest Anim*, 46, 664-673.

[44] Rigau, T., Farré, M., Ballester, J., Mogas, T., Peña, A., & Rodríguez-Gil, J. E. (2001). Effects of glucose and fructose on motility patterns of dog spermatozoa from fresh ejaculates. *Theriogenology*, 56, 801-815.

[45] Rigau, T., Rivera, M., Palomo-Novell, M. J., Fernández., J. M., Mogas, T., Ballester, J., Peña, A., Otaegui, P. J., Guinovart, J. J., & Rodríguez-Gil, J. E. (2002). Differential effects of glucose and fructose on hexose metabolism in dog spermatozoa. *Reproduction*, 123, 579-591.

[46] Rodríguez- Gil, J. E. (2006). Mammalian sperm energy resources management and survival during conservation in refrigeration. *Reprod Domest Anim*, 41(2), 11-20.

[47] Salisbury, G. W., VanDemark, N. L., & Lodge, J. R. (1978). Sperm survival into the female reproductive tract. *In: Physiology of reproduction and artificial insemination of cattle. Salisbury GW, VanDemark NL, Lodge JR, eds*, 394-396, WH Freeman and Co., San Francisco (USA).

[48] Setchell, B. P., & Brooks, D. E. (1994). Seminal plasma. *In: The Physiology of Reproduction. Knobil E, Neill JD, eds.*, 797-836, Raven Press, 0-88167-281-5, York (USA).

[49] Schlegel, W., Rotermund, S., Färber, G., & Nieschlag, E. (1981). The influence of prostaglandins on sperm motility. *Prostaglandins*, 21, 87-99.

[50] Storey, B. T., & Kayne, F. J. (1978). Energy metabolism of spermatozoa. VII. Interactions between lactate, pyruvate and malate as oxidative substrates for rabbit sperm mitochondria. *Biol Reprod*, 18, 527-536.

[51] Suarez, S. S., & Ho, H. C. (2003). Hyperactivated motility in sperm. *Reprod Domest Anim*, 38, 119-124.

[52] Templeton, A. A., Cooper, I., & Kelly, R. W. (1978). Prostaglandin concentrations in the semen of fertile men. *J Reprod Fertil*, 52, 147-150.

[53] Visconti, P. E., Galantino-Homer, H., Moore, G. D., Bailey, J. I., Ning, T. X., Fornes, M., & Kopf, G. S. (1998). The molecular basis of sperm capacitation. *J Androl*, 19, 242-248.

[54] Visconti, P. E. (2009). Understanding the molecular basis of sperm capacitation through kinase design. Proc Nat Am Soc USA , 106, 667-688.

[55] Yanagimachi, R. (1994). Mammalian fertilization. In: The Physiology of Reproduction. Knobil E, Neil JD, eds. 189-317, *Raven Press, Ltd., 2nd ed. New York (USA).*

[56] Yang, W. C., Kwok, S. C. M., Leshin, S., Bollo, E., & Li, W. I. (1998). Purified porcine seminal plasma protein enhances in vitro immune activities of porcine peripheral lymphocytes. *Biol Reprod*, 59, 202-207.

Chapter 10

Artificial Insemination in Poultry

M.R. Bakst and J.S. Dymond

Additional information is available at the end of the chapter

http://dx.doi.org/10.5772/54918

1. Introduction

Artificial insemination (AI) is the manual transfer of semen into the female's vagina. Basically it is a two step procedure: first, collecting semen from the male [1]; and second, inseminating the semen into the female [2]. In poultry, depending on the objectives and goals of the farm or laboratory, there may be intervening steps such as semen dilution, storage, and evaluation.

Artificial insemination is practiced extensively with commercial turkeys. This is primarily the result of selective breeding for a heavier and broader-breasted commercial turkey and the consequent inability of toms to consistently transfer semen to the hen at copulation. The broiler industry has not adapted AI to the extent of the turkey industry but it is occasionally used in pedigree lines and in regions where labor is relatively cheap.

To grasp the magnitude of AI in the turkey industry compared to that of livestock, a hypothetical flock of 500 breeder hens inseminated with 100 μL of diluted semen (1:1) twice the week before the onset of egg production and once weekly thereafter for the 24 wk of egg production would entail 13,000 inseminations using 650 mL of semen. It should be apparent with these numbers, semen collection and hen inseminations are labor intensive as each male and female must be handled each week.

Looking back over the use of AI in the turkey industry one can safely say that in the 1960s, weekly inseminations were based on semen volume per dose using undiluted semen. In the 1970s and early 1980s, breeder farms began to dilute semen and inseminate a known number of sperm per dose. In the mid-1980s through the 1990s, hens were initially inseminated a week before the onset of lay and inseminations were performed with a known number of 'viable' sperm. Currently, while inseminating before the onset of egg production remains widely practiced, most companies, but not all [3], have gone back to inseminating a known volume of semen or number of sperm per dose, in the 1970s and 1980s.

In the following chapter we will review the basics of AI and fertility evaluation in poultry. To better appreciate the biological basis of these techniques, an overview of the reproductive biology of poultry is provided. Detailed descriptions of techniques for the collection, evaluation, dilution, and storage of poultry semen are available in a recent publication by Bakst and Long [4]. Earlier comprehensive reviews include Lake and Stewart [5], Bakst and Wishart [6], and Bakst and Cecil [7].

2. Reproductive biology of poultry

This section will introduce to some and review for others the strategy of avian reproduction with emphasis on the hen. For more comprehensive reviews on reproduction in the avian male and female see Jamieson [8].

2.1. Overview

The goal of AI is to produce a succession of fertilized eggs between successive inseminations. To accomplish this, weekly inseminations must replenish the sperm population in the uterovaginal junction (UVJ) sperm storage tubules (SSTs). Birds do not have an estrous cycle that synchronizes copulation with ovulation. Alternatively, about 7-10 days before their first ovulation, hens mate, sperm ascend the vagina and then enter the SSTs. At the onset of egg production, individual sperm are slowly released from the SSTs, transported to the anterior end of the oviduct, and interact with the surface of the ovum (see [9-10] for recent reviews). Whether fertilized or not, over the next 24-26 hr the ovum is transported though the oviduct, accruing the outer perivitelline layer (PL) in the infundibulum, the albumen in the magnum, the shell membrane in the isthmus, and the hard shell in the uterus (also referred to as the shell gland) before oviposition. If fertilized, the blastoderm in the first laid egg consists of 40,000-60,000 cells in the turkey and 80,000-100,000 cells in the chicken.

Ovary: In the hen only the left ovary and oviduct become functional organs. About 2-3 wk before the onset of lay, small (less than 1 mm in diameter) white-yolk follicles begin to accumulate yellow yolk with some being recruited into a hierarchy of maturing yellow-yolk follicles (Figure 1). At the time of ovulation, the largest follicle, designated as F1, is ovulated. About 17 days were necessary for the 1 mm diameter white yolk follicle to mature to a pre-ovulatory 40 mm diameter yellow yolk follicle [11]. After the F1 follicle is ovulated, the next largest follicle, formerly designated F2, becomes the F1 follicle and will ovulate at the beginning of the next daily "ovulatory cycle" in 24-26 hr.

The follicular sheath surrounding the maturing oocyte consists of histologically distinct concentric layers of cells: the outer serosa (germinal epithelium); the theca externa, which forms the greatest portion of the follicle wall, provides structural support to the follicle and has steriodogenic cells; the theca interna, a highly vascularized layer, which like the theca externa has steroid-producing cells (both thecal layers synthesize androgens and estrogens); and, the granulosa cell layer, enveloping the oocyte, which is responsible for progesterone secretion and the synthesis of the inner PL. The inner PL is homologous to the mammalian zona pellucida and

http://dx.doi.org/10.5772/54918

is a fibrous reticulum about 2 μm thick. At ovulation, only the inner PL envelops the ovum. While there is no corpus luteum formation in birds, the thecal layers and the granulosa of the post-ovulatory follicle (POF) produce prostaglandins [12] and progesterone, respectively [13-16] then regress over the next 72 hr. The POF has a pocket like appearance after ovulation (Figure 1). On the surface of the inner PL overlying the germinal disc (GD), which is a 3.5 mm diameter disc of white yolk containing the haploid pronucleus and associated organelles, are sperm receptors. Sperm bind to the receptors overlying the GD, hydrolyze a path through the inner PL, and are incorporated into the ovum. Polyspermy is normal in birds but only one sperm in apposition to the female pronucleus undergoes nuclear decondensation and initiates syngamy, the reconstitution of the diploid number of chromosomes.

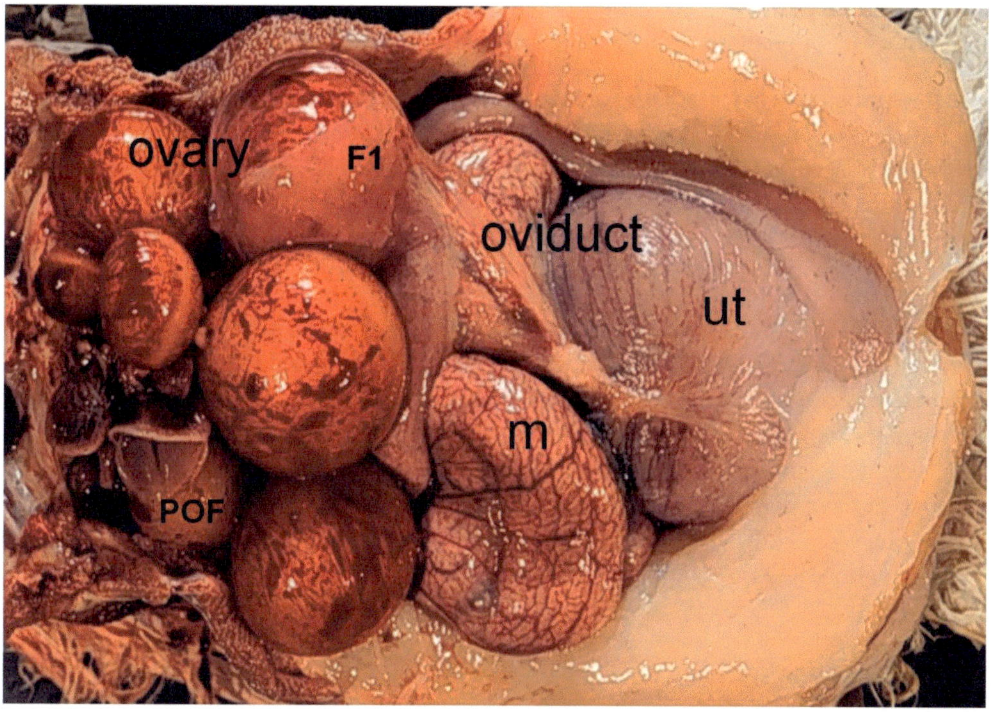

Figure 1. The ovary and oviduct of a turkey hen in egg production occupy much of the abdominal cavity. The ovarian follicular hierarchy consisting of ovarian follicles at various stages of develop (7 maturing follicles visible in this photograph) is observed. The largest follicle, F1 follicle is the next to ovulate. The ovum ovulated about 10 hr earlier has accrued albumen in the magnum (m), a shell membrane in the isthmus, and is observed in the uterus (ut) undergoing shell formation. Its post-ovulatory follicular sheath (POF) appears as an open pocket. The vagina (distal to the uterus and not visible) is embedded in connective tissue and enveloped by the abdominal fat pad.

2.2. Oviduct

The mature oviduct consists of five anatomically and functionally distinct segments (Figures 1 and 2): the infundibulum, which secretes an albumen-like product that forms the outer PL and prevents pathological polyspermy; the magnum, responsible for deposition of the albumen proteins; the isthmus, which forms the shell membrane; the uterus (also referred to as the shell gland), a pocket-like structure that elaborates the hard-shell; and, the vagina, which is a conduit between the uterus and cloaca for the egg-mass at oviposition and is responsible for sperm selection and storage following semen transfer. Interestingly, when the vagina and uterus are excised and fixed *in toto* and the connective tissue surrounding the vagina subsequently removed, the vagina appears as a coiled segment (Figure 3) [10]. This anatomy explains the resistance one feels when performing a vaginal insemination with a straw regardless of the presence or absence of an egg mass in the uterus. If inseminating a hen within 30 min after oviposition, the connective tissue around the vagina and the smooth muscle composing the vaginal wall are flaccid. Venting (exteriorizing the vagina for placement of the inseminating straw) at this time may induce a partial prolapse leading to a deep insemination (closer to the UVJ) and the forfeiture of sperm selection by the vagina. Such deep inseminations are associated with high embryo mortality, possibly due to pathological polyspermy.

The surface mucosa of each segment of the oviduct is lined with parallel, gently spiraling folds along the longitudinal axis. The surface epithelium lining the luminal mucosa contains varying proportions of secretory and ciliated cells. All segments except the fimbriated region of the infundibulum and the vagina possess sub-epithelial tubular glands that secrete components used in egg formation [17]. However, the anterior 2-3 cm of the vagina, an area referred to as the UVJ (Figure 3), contains the SSTs, the primary sites of sperm storage [10] (Figure 4).

At ovulation, the ovum is grasped by the fimbriated region of the infundibulum and, if sperm are present, the ovum may be fertilized within a 10-15 min interval [18]. Thereafter, infundibular secretions accrue around the ovum, forming the outer PL, which acts as a barrier to further sperm penetration. Birkhead [19] observed that the number of sperm trapped in the outer PL is positively correlated with the size of the ovum and is likewise correlated with the number of sperm that have penetrated the inner PL. Interestingly, the sperm trapped in the outer PL retain an intact acrosome [20-21]. If fertilized, the first cleavage furrow in the GD appears 7-8 hr post-ovulation, while the egg-mass is in the isthmus.

2.3. Oviductal sperm selection, transport, and storage

Following deposition in the oviduct, sperm are transported to UVJ by a combination of their intrinsic motility and cilia beat activity [9-10, 22-23]. Within the SST lumen, sperm are either widely spaced or oriented parallel with their heads toward the distal end of the SST (Figure 4). Sperm are apposed to, but not directly contacting the apical microvilli of the SST epithelial cells. This spatial relationship may facilitate lipid transfer between the resident sperm and the SST epithelial cells [24-25]. Interestingly, alkaline phosphatase, known to play a role in lipid transfer, has been histochemically localized in the apical region of the SST epithelium [26].

The duration of sperm storage in the SSTs is species-dependent. Chickens can store sperm for up to three weeks, whereas turkeys can maintain sperm for 10 weeks in the SST and still lay a fertilized ovum [27-28]. This may be related to number of SSTs present in the UVJ; turkeys have been reported to have 20,000-30,000 SSTs, while chickens have been estimated to have only 5,000-13,500 [29-30]. Additionally, after several generations of selection for high fertility, chicken hens possessed increased numbers of SSTs when compared to non-selected control hens, suggesting the number of SSTs may be positively correlated with fertility [31]. In contrast, under commercial conditions, different broiler strains exhibiting different fertility levels revealed similar numbers of SSTs [29].

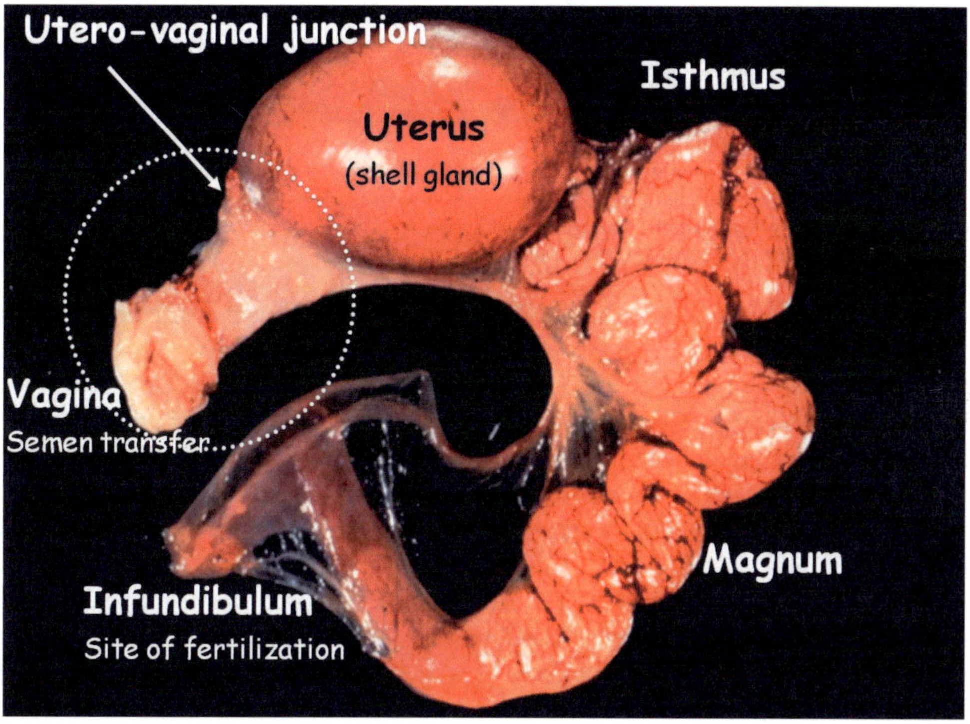

Figure 2. The segments of the turkey oviduct with a hard-shelled egg in the uterus are observed. Sperm transferred into the vagina undergo an intense selection process before reaching the sperm storage tubules (SSTs) localized in the utero-vaginal junction. Sperm are slowly released from the SSTs and ascend to the infundibulum, the site of fertilization. In this photograph, the vagina is enveloped by connective tissue.

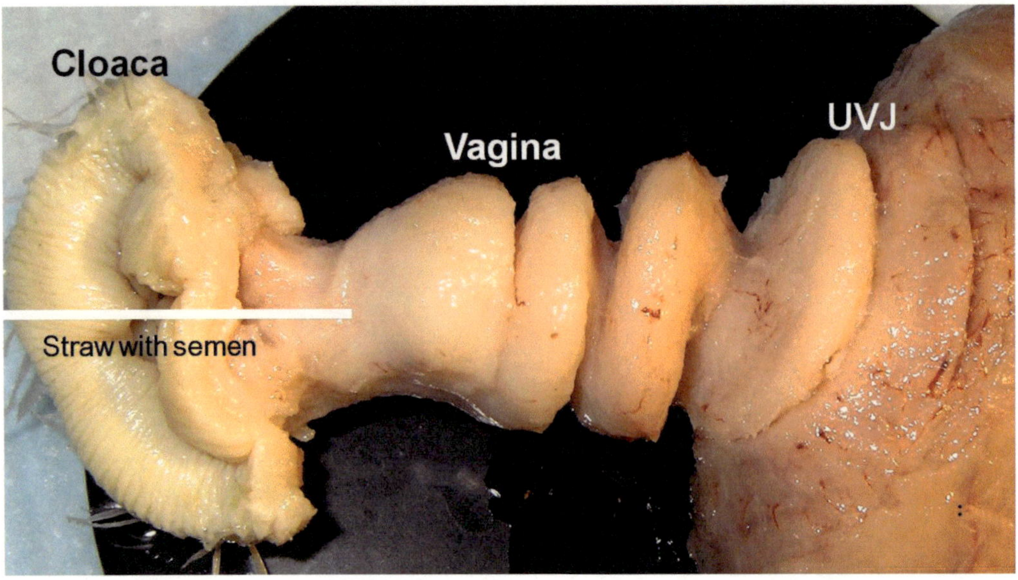

Figure 3. Following fixation in neutral-buffered formalin and the removal of the surrounding connective tissue, the coiled morphology of the turkey vagina is revealed. When inseminating a hen, one should insert the straw with the semen until resistance is felt, then release the semen as the straw is withdrawn. As observed here the resistance is due to the coiled vaginal and not an egg mass in the uterus.

Little is known concerning the cellular and molecular mechanisms that sustain sperm within the SST lumen for prolonged periods of storage. These mechanisms likely involve the reversible suppression of sperm motility and metabolism, protection and repair of the sperm plasma membrane, uptake and storage of molecules to sustain sperm metabolism, and maintenance of the SST lumen by removing by-products of sperm metabolism and degraded sperm [32-33]. It is clear the SSTs generate a discrete environment to maintain sperm viability via the influx and efflux of compounds critical for sperm survival [25, 34). While ultrastructural analysis has revealed only limited evidence of secretory activity [25], the identification of membrane-bound vesicles released from the apical tips of the SST epithelial cell microvilli suggests a role in the maintenance of resident sperm through lipid transfer [22, 25, 26, 32, 35, 36]. A large proportion of the sperm plasma membrane is composed of polyunsaturated fatty acids [37] that are highly susceptible to damage induced by lipid peroxidation [37]. The peroxidation of these fatty acids results in increased damage to and permeability of the sperm plasma membrane [39, 40]. A complex system of anti-oxidation enzymes are present in the SST epithelial cells and presumably interact with luminal sperm to minimize damage due to lipid peroxidation and maintain sperm membrane integrity [41]. While many metabolites required by sperm in the SSTs have yet to be identified, increased avidin expression is apparent in SSTs relative to surrounding UVJ epithelial tissue possibly providing a means of sequestering biotin and other vitamins for use by the SSTs or resident sperm [42-43]. Interestingly, progesterone has been shown to induce expression of avidin in the oviduct, providing a potential link between progesterone fluctuation and sperm storage in and release from the SSTs [42, 44, 45].

http://dx.doi.org/10.5772/54918

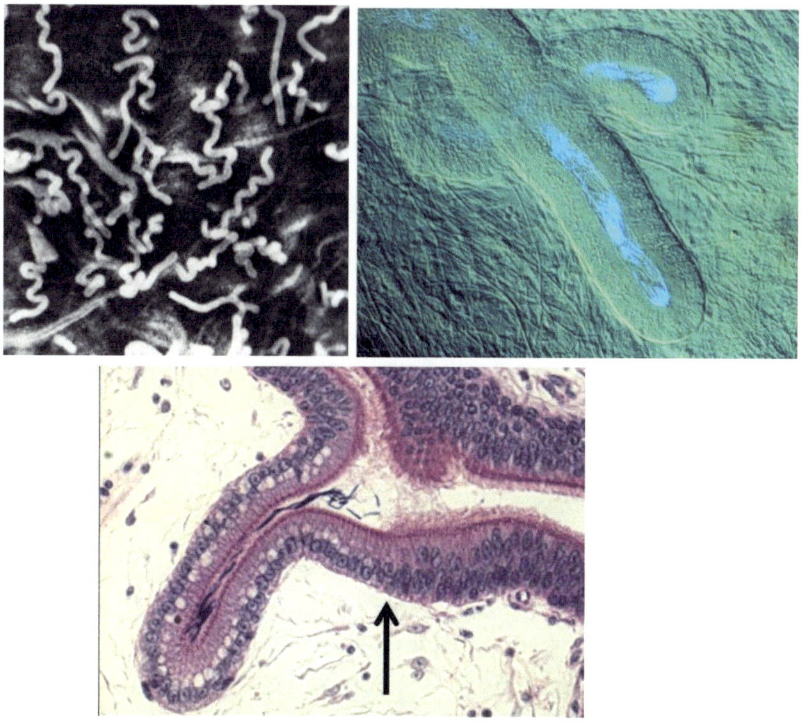

Figure 4. Three views of the turkey's sperm-storage tubules (SSTs) are observed. The left panel is a stereoscope image showing the pleomorphic appearance of the SSTs. The length of the SST can be as long as 300µm. In the right panel a hen was inseminated with sperm stained with Hoechst 33342, a nuclear fluorescent dye, the UVJ mucosa containing SSTs was isolated, and an unfixed squash preparation was observed by dual interference contrast and fluorescence microscopy. Sperm with fluorescing nuclei are observed in the two SST lumina. The lower-middle panel shows a histological section of a portion of a SST containing sperm (the dense rod-like structures in the lumen are sperm nuclei. The arrow indicates the transition between the pseudo-stratified columnar ciliated epithelium of the uterovaginal junction and the simple columnar epithelium of the SST that is characterized in histological preparations by the supra-nuclear vacuole.

Sperm exit the SSTs in a slow, continuous stream [46-49]; however, a stimulus cuing the egress of resident sperm from the SSTs has yet to be identified. The observations that receptors for estrogen and progesterone exist in the SSTs has led to the suggestion that these compounds may trigger release of resident sperm, possibly in response to hormonal cues over the course of the ovulatory cycle[50-52]. However, an alternate theory suggests the inherent mobility of the sperm plays a larger role than hormonal induction in egress of sperm from SSTs [9]. Resident sperm exhibit a slow, synchronized oscillatory movement in the lumen of SSTs, suggesting the presence of a fluid current through the SST lumen [23-24]. The identification of water channels, known as aquaporins, in the apical epithelium of SSTs lends credence to a model wherein motile sperm maintain their residence in the SST lumen by swimming against the fluid current generated via the aquaporins [53-56]. In the SST lumen, sperm retain their motility by fatty acid oxidation. It has been suggested the sperm membrane is the source of this fatty acid and that as the quality of the sperm membrane gradually decreases there is a reduction of available ATP and sperm motility decreases [56]. Sperm are then swept out of the SST lumen into the UVJ, where they encounter various stimuli enhancing their motility. These sperm are then transported to the infundibulum, the site of fertilization [57]. Such motility-enhancing factors may include changes in environmental pH and neuroendocrine factors such as serotonin [58-62]. Further oxidation of sperm fatty acids, possibly sequestered from the surround milieu, generates the energy required for sperm to respond to such motility-enhancing factors and transcend the oviduct [9, 22, 55, 63].

Once sperm are deposited in the oviduct, several selection barriers must be overcome prior to ascending to the infundibulum and fertilizing an ovum. This selection occurs initially in the vagina: only highly mobile (defined as progressive movement in a viscous medium at 40°C) sperm traverse the vagina [9]. While sperm mobility is a major factor in sperm selection in the vagina, sperm selection is also dependent upon the glycoprotein composition of the sperm plasma membrane. The sperm glycocalyx is highly complex and heavily sialylated and modification of the glycocalyx results in reduced fertility and failure of the sperm to enter the SSTs [64-67]. Interestingly, removal of membrane-associated carbohydrates did not affect sperm entry into SSTs if sperm were inseminated directly into the UVJ or when co-incubated with UVJ explants, suggesting the glycocalyx plays a central role in sperm transport and selection through the vagina [64, 66, 68]. Further barriers to sperm prior participating in the process of fertilization include sperm release from the SST and subsequent transport to the infundibulum, and their interaction with the ovum (reviewed in [69]).

2.4. Sperm: Ovum interaction and fertilization

Given the voluminous nature of the hen's ovum and the GD relative to mammalian ova, one must assume that yet-to-be identified factors "attract" sperm to the GD. Examination of the electrophoretic profile of the GD and non-GD regions of the PL revealed no variation in protein composition [70]. Furthermore, the abrogation of the preferential interaction of sperm and the inner PL overlying the GD *in vitro* suggests the factors underlying the preferential binding of sperm are not necessarily associated with the inner PL [70]. It is clear, however, glycoproteins play a large role in the interaction between the sperm and ova, even if not directly involved in targeting of sperm to the GD *in vivo* [71]. Pre-treatment of either the PL or sperm with N-glycanases resulted in significantly decreased sperm-ovum interaction *in vitro* [68, 71]. Conversely, N-linked oligosaccharides released from the inner PL by N-glycosidase treatment could induce the acrosome reaction in sperm *in vitro* [72]. These findings strongly suggest N-linked glycans, most likely terminal N-acetyl glucosamine residues, have an essential role in the sperm-ovum interaction in avian species, specifically in induction of the acrosome reaction [68, 72].

Interaction between the sperm and inner PL results in induction of the acrosome reaction [73]. During the acrosome reaction, the inner and outer acrosomal membranes dehisce resulting in the release of acrosin (a trypsin-like enzyme) [21, 74]. As the result of the acrosome reaction, sperm hydrolyze a small hole in the inner PL (Figure 5), enabling sperm to reach the microvilli-studded surface of the ovum [21, 74]. The capacity of sperm to hydrolyze and penetrate the inner PL is the biological basis for the sperm penetration assay discussed below and next section.

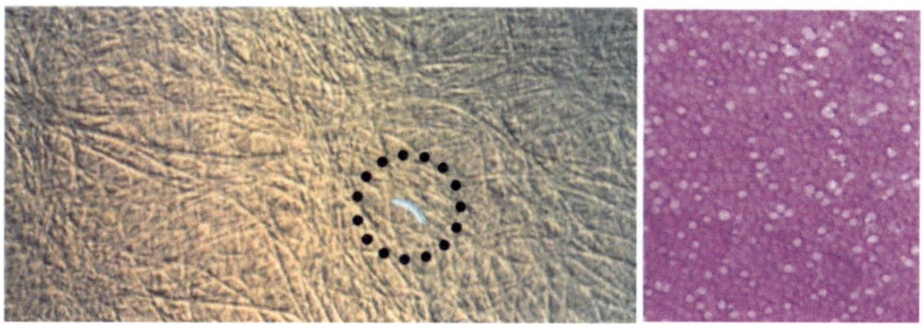

Figure 5. In the left panel, a turkey sperm stained with Hoechst 33342 prior to insemination is observed on the surface of the inner perivitelline layer (PL). The sperm's acrosome will release a trypsin like enzyme, acrosin, and digest a hole through the inner PL. The right panel shows multiple sperm holes (white perforations) in the inner PL overlying the germinal disc (GD) of a duck ovum (polyspermy is normal in birds). Sperm hole numbers can be used to assess true fertility and the duration of the fertile period..

Unlike mammals, polyspermy is the norm in avian fertilization. The GD (3.5 mm in diameter) provides a relatively small target for fertilization in the large megalecithal ova (yolk-filled ova) of chickens and turkeys (3.5 – 4.0 mm in diameter); thus polyspermy may be an evolutionary adaptation to ensure higher rates of fertilization in such species [74]. The inner PL may be penetrated by many sperm, although only one male pronucleus will ultimately fuse (syngamy) with the female pronucleus to form the nascent embryo (reviewed in [75-77]. A single sperm hole in the inner PL does not ensure fertilization. Although turkeys show a lower number of sperm interacting with ova relative to chickens, the presence of three sperm holes in the inner PL predicts a 50% probability of fertilization, whereas, six sperm holes suggest a probability greater than 95% fertilization [78]. The outer PL is rapidly depositied around the ovum in the posterior infundibulum and proximal magnum and is impenetrable by sperm [21, 78-79] thus preventing pathological polyspermy.

Given the volume of the GD relative to a single sperm, another possible function of polyspermy may be to activate specific molecular factors in the GD cytoplasm thereby initiating the process of embryogenesis. Yet, polyspermy also results in the presence of multiple male pronuclei in the GD. To cope with this potentially harmful scenario, the mature ovum has been found to have DNase I and II endonuclease activities, both of which will degrade sperm DNA [76]. In contrast, no such DNase activity has been detected in mammalian ova that engage in monospermic fertilization, further suggesting the role of these enzymes in the avian embryo is to protect against detrimental genetic consequences of polyspermy [76].

The number of holes in the inner PL is highly positively correlated with fertility. Correlations exist between the number of sperm inseminated, the number undergoing the acrosome reaction at the inner PL [80], and the number of sperm embedded in the outer PL [81]. The number of sperm holes in the inner PL and the number sperm trapped in the outer PL may be used to estimate the duration of fertility ('fertile period') in hens. While the number of sperm penetrating the inner PL shows a decreasing logarithmic relationship over time [81-82], a positive correlation between the total number of sperm penetrating the inner PL and the number of sperm stored in the SSTs was observed [83]. Given these observations, it should not be surprising there is also a positive correlation between the number of SSTs containing sperm and the proportion of sperm that have undergone the acrosome reaction at the inner PL [82].

3. Techniques in artificial insemination and fertility evaluation in poultry

For non-domestic birds, chapters in Bakst and Long [4], Lake and Stewart [5] and Bakst and Wishart [6] provide overviews of semen evaluation and AI techniques. Artificial insemination technology and reproductive biology for ratites were reviewed by Malecki et al. [84].

3.1. Semen collection

Primarily due to the anatomical variation of the phallic region in different birds, semen collection techniques will vary. In contrast to ratites and water-fowl with an intromittent phallus, Galliformes (chicken, turkey, and quail) do not have an intermittent organ. Their non-intromittent organ consists of folds and bulges that make contact with the female's cloaca at mating. From an anatomical perspective, there are considerable differences between the non-intromittent organs of the chicken and turkey (Figure 6). The rooster has a prominent medial phallic body and relatively small lateral phallic bodies and lymph folds. Conversely, the turkey tom has no medial phallic body but prominent lateral phallic bodies and lymph folds. Sex sorting at hatch by cloacal examination is based on the relative differences in size of these structures between the males and females.

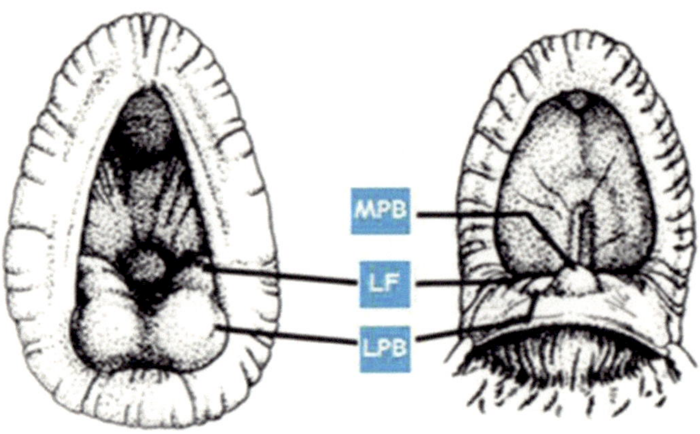

Figure 6. The turkey (left) and chicken (right) cloacae are viewed with the dorsal lips of the cloacae pulled back to expose each species phallus non-protrudens. Unlike the turkey, the chicken has a central protuberance, the medial phallic body (MPB) and regressed lateral phallic bodies (LPB) and lymph folds (LF). The turkey phallus non-protrudens is characterized by dominant LPB and LF and the conspicuous absence of the MPB.

The goal of semen collector is to obtain the maximum volume of clean, high quality semen with the minimal amount of handling. In chickens and turkeys, the abdominal massage technique [1, 4] involves massaging the cloacal region to achieve phallic tumescence. This is followed by a 'cloacal stroke', a squeezing of the region surrounding the sides of the cloaca to express the semen. Little additional semen can be expressed after two cloacal strokes; additional cloacal strokes may cause damage to the phallic and cloacal regions and contribute to semen contamination [85].

Semen should be pearly white, viscous, and clean. With each male collected, the semen collector should perform a visual examination of the semen at the time of ejaculation. This is easier with the turkey because the ejaculate accumulates on the phallus before it is collected by the 'milker' (semen collector). Off-color or watery semen, and semen contaminated with blood or fecal/urates debris should not be used for insemination. Due to the increased volume of transparent fluid in rooster semen, which is a transudate derived from the phallus at the time of ejaculation, chicken semen is less viscous and sperm concentration lower than that of turkey semen.

3.2. Sperm concentration

If semen is to be diluted, it is best .to have a known volume of semen diluent (a tissue culture-like medium formulated to sustain sperm viability) at ambient temperature in the semen receptacle before collection begins. For routine AI of turkey hens, semen from 10-12 toms are pooled in a single receptacle, mixing the semen gently after each male is collected. Semen volume is determined and if the AI dose is based on numbers of sperm (generally 250-350 million sperm per dose) sperm concentration is determined. The most popular techniques for determining sperm concentration are the packed cell volume (PCV; also referred to as a spermatocrit) and optical density (OD; photometry).

Determining sperm concentration using PCVs is nearly identical to that of determining blood hematocrit values. Semen aspirated into micro-hematocrit tubes are centrifuged in a hematocrit centrifuge until the sperm are tightly packed (10 min); the percentage of packed sperm cells relative to the original semen volume in the micro-tube is determined. Sperm concentration is derived using a conversion factor or standard curve previously derived by comparing and graphically plotting varying ascending sperm concentrations from hemocytometer counts to corresponding spermatocrit readings. (See [4] for detailed protocols to determine sperm concentration and the derivation of standard curves.)

The optical density (OD) is determined using a photometer. The OD of highly diluted semen is directly proportional to the concentration of sperm, thus providing an indirect estimate of the sperm concentration. Like the PCV method, sperm concentration is derived using a conversion factor or previously derived standard curve by comparing and graphically plotting varying sperm concentrations from hemocytometer counts to corresponding OD readings [4].

The PVC and OD methods are two *indirect* methods of determining sperm concentration, that is, the final concentration is calculated from a regression equation or standard curve derived, in part, from *direct* sperm counts with a hemocytometer [4]. Briefly, to derive a regression equation and standard curve, serial dilutions (n=5) covering a wide range of sperm concentrations are prepared and sperm concentrations are determined with a hemocytometer and the instrument or method that requires the standard curve (at least 4 replicates with 4 different semen samples). This is a tedious procedure but if reliable and repeatable sperm numbers are to be inseminated it is best to establish standard curves for each instrument every 12-18 months. The reason for this is that the rotational speed of different centrifuges and the intensity of a photometer's light source may differ as a result of manufacturer's variation, age of the instrument, and/or repeated use of the instrument, thereby producing variations in the respective final readings and subsequent calculations of sperm concentrations.

Another concern when using any semen evaluation method is variation in the operator's techniques. Consistency is the key to repeatable data. The technical staff all must follow the same standard operating procedures (SOPs). For example, when counting sperm with a hemocytometer, all individuals in a lab should following the same SOP for how long the sperm are permitted to settle on the grid and which sperm to count or omit from the count. Also, is the photometer zeroed with the same buffer? If a procedure calls for an incubation period, such as in a live-dead stain, are the samples being incubated for the same duration each time using the same stain concentrations? A lack of consistency in following the SOPs within a laboratory will lead to unwarranted variation and non-reproducible and inaccurate data.

3.3. Sperm viability

In the context of semen evaluation, reference to 'viable' sperm simply implies that such sperm possess an intact plasmalemma and are assumed to be functional. Plasmalemma integrity is frequently determined using either a dead-cell or a live-cell stain alone or simultaneously. The dead-cell stains are excluded by sperm with an intact plasmalemma but stain dead sperm possessing a permeable plasmalemma. Live-cell stains permeate the intact sperm plasmalemma and become visible only after reacting with cytosolic enzymes or interacting with sperm nuclear proteins. Both eosin and propidium iodide are popular dead-cell stains while calcein AM and SYBR-14 are frequently used live-cell stains (see [86] for extended discussion and availability for the live-cell probes). On a commercial breeder farm, the nigrosin/eosin (N/E) technique is most likely the procedure to be used to determine sperm viability [4]. Briefly, sperm are stained with N/E and a smear of the stained sperm is made on a slide (Figure 7). Under a bright field microscope the viable sperm remain pearly white, while eosin will stain non-viable sperm a pink to magenta color. The nigrosin serves as a background to enhance differentiation between the non-viable and viable sperm. In contrast to the N/E technique, a more sophisticated laboratory may use flow cytometry that sorts viable from non-viable sperm after staining with calcein AM or SYBR-14 and propidium iodide.

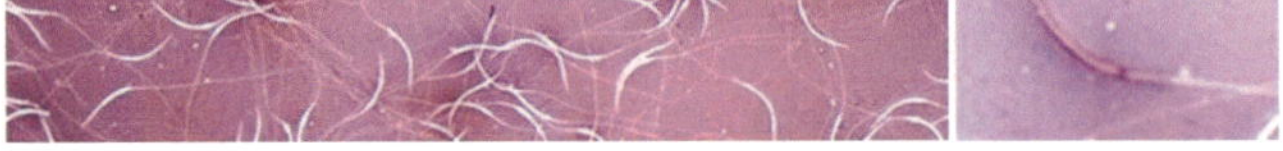

Figure 7. The left panel shows a nigrosin eosin preparation of turkey sperm with nearly 100% viable sperm (unstained) white nuclei and midpieces. The sperm head is clearly visible as the white arcing segment; the acrosome and midpiece are difficult to differentiate from the nucleus. The upper right panel reveals a normal sperm and a second sperm with an abnormally curved and swollen midpiece. Observed in the lower right panel is a nonviable sperm stained with eosin throughout the nucleus and midpiece. Barely visible at the anterior end of the nucleus is the unstained, conical shaped acrosome.

3.4. Sperm motility and mobility

Sperm motility can be progressive (forward direction) or non-progressive (random movement or oscillations) movement. Generally, progressive motility is determined subjectively at ambient temperature using a microscope at low magnification (hanging-drop technique) or objectively using a computer-assisted semen analysis system. These techniques are reviewed by Bakst and Long [4]. Motility evaluated by microscopy has been shown to have little correlation with fertility and simply reveals that the sperm are motile. First described by Froman and McLean [87] and further elaborated for commercial use by Froman [88], the sperm mobility assay has gained popularity as a measure of an individual male's ability to produce highly mobile sperm [mobility defines the ability of sperm to move progressively against a viscous medium (Accudenz) at 41°C] that are more likely to fertilize an ovum than males producing less mobile sperm. While the sperm mobility assay is a powerful tool for the selection of the most fecund males to be used in AI, it necessitates attention to details and accurate and consistent preparation of the reagents.

3.5. Evaluation of fertility

The measure of a successful AI program is sustained hen fertility. While candling-fertility is useful, there is an eight or more day lag between the last AI and candling-fertility determination, which overlaps with the next insemination (hen insemination is generally at 7-day intervals). With AI programs, it is often desirable to determine the fertility status of a flock before the next weekly insemination. There are several options available: breaking-out fresh eggs and examining the GD to differentiate a fertilized from an unfertilized or early dead embryo; setting normal but culled eggs (checked, hairline cracked, or dirty eggs) in a spare incubator for 24-36 hr before breaking-out [89]; counting sperm in the outer PL; and counting sperm holes in the inner PL. The above procedures are reviewed in Bakst and Long [4].

As noted previously, the sperm penetration assay is not only used to determine true fertility, but also to estimate the number of sperm residing in the use SSTs at the time of ovulation [90]. The isolation of the inner PL and staining procedure, initially developed for chicken eggs by Bramwell et al. [91], was quickly adapted to turkey eggs by Donoghue [92]. The major drawback to the sperm penetration assay as originally described is that it is time consuming, particularly with respect to isolating, washing, and positioning the PL wrinkle-free on the slide. Spasojevic [10] and colleagues at Willmar Poultry Company (Willmar, MN) significantly increased the efficiency of preparing the PL slides from turkey eggs in the following manner: the albumen is removed from the ovum as in the original procedure [4]; a square is outlined on a slide using super glue; the slide is placed firmly on the ovum's surface with the GD centered in the square; after the glue is set, the PL is cut and washed to remove adhering yolk. The advantages here are speed and the PL remains wrinkle free.

A different modification of the sperm penetration assay was suggested by I.A. Malecki (personal communication) and entails placing a filter ring over the GD (inside diameter slightly larger than the GD), cutting around the outside diameter of the filter ring (about 2 mm between the inside and outside perimeter of the ring), and lifting the filter ring off the ovum. The filter ring with the adhering PL is washed gently with saline to remove the yolk and GD material until transparent, placed on a slide, and then fixed and stained with saline washes after each step. Our laboratory has used the filter ring technique with eggs from broilers, turkeys, ducks, and quail and it is now our preferred method for the performing the sperm penetration assay.

4. Conclusion

Artificial insemination is a common practice in the poultry industry with the turkey industry in North America and Europe using it almost exclusively for the production of hatching eggs. The broiler industry has not adapted AI for several reasons: because of sheer numbers of broiler breeders that need to be inseminated weekly, the labor cost would be very significantly; the initial investment in special housing for the males; an efficient, cost effective means of actually performing the inseminations (housing and catching the hens) would need to be developed; and finally, the concern that after a few generations of breeding broilers by AI, the behaviors associated with natural mating may be less dominant. Notwithstanding these concerns, the benefits of AI for broilers would include the following: the male:female ratio would be increase from 1:10 for natural mating to 1:25 with AI; with fewer males needed, there would be greater selection pressure on the male traits of economic importance and subsequently greater genetic advancement per generation; biosecurity concerns associated with "spiking" aging hen flocks with new and/or younger males to augment mating frequency and fertility would be eliminated; and, differences in body conformation between males and females that impact semen transfer at mating would no longer be a consideration.

In 1995, Sir Peter Lake wrote an excellent review of the history of AI, its impact on the poultry industry, and what is needed to advance the practice of AI with poultry [93]. Unfortunately, AI technology has not advanced significant since this review article. More than 15 years later, the only significant advance is in the evaluation of sperm mobility and the impact that males producing highly mobile sperm have on paternity [9]. Notwithstanding, it is foreseeable that sometime in the future, research addressing poultry sperm biology and the cellular and molecular basis of oviductal sperm transport, selection, and storage will lead to the following innovations in AI technology: insemination intervals increased to 10-14 days (versus 7-day) with fewer sperm per insemination; *in vitro* sperm storage for 24-36 hr at ambient temperature with minimal loss of sperm viability; and, the possibility of transgenic progeny following the insemination of sperm carrying transgenes.

Author details

M.R. Bakst* and J.S. Dymond

*Address all correspondence to: murray.bakst@ars.usda.gov

Animal Biosciences and Biotechnology Laboratory Beltsville Area, Agricultural Research Service, U.S. Department of Agriculture Beltsville, Maryland, USA

References

[1] Burrows WA, Quinn JP. The method of obtaining spermatoza from the domestic fowl. Poultry Science 1935;14(4) 251-4.

[2] Quinn JP, Burrows WA. Artificial insemination in fowls. The Journal of Heredity 1936;27(1) 31-7.

[3] Spasojevic R. Two hundred million sperm cells per hen? No Way! *Proceedings – Midwest Poultry Federation Convention*, Turkey Breeder Workshop, March 16-18, 2010. CD available at MPF. St. Paul, Minnesota. www.midwestpoultry.com

[4] Bakst MR, Long JA. Techniques for Semen Evaluation, Semen Storage, and Fertility Determination. 2, 1-113. 2010. St. Paul, Minnesota, The Midwest Poultry Federation.

[5] Lake PE, Stewart JM. Artificial insemination in poultry. Bulletin 213. 1978. London, UK, Ministry of Agriculture, Fish, and Food. Her Majesty's Stationary Office.

[6] Bakst MR, Wishart GJ. Proceedings, First Internation Symposium on the Artificial Insemination of Poultry. 1, 1-297. 1995. Champaign, IL, Poultry Science Association, Inc.

[7] Bakst MR, Cecil H. Techniques for Semen Evaluation, Semen Storage, and Fertility Determination. 1-97. 1997. Savoy, IL, Poultry Science Association.

[8] Jamieson BGM. Reproductive Biology and Phylogeny of Birds. Enfield, New Hampshire: Science Publishers; 2007.

[9] Froman DP, Feltmann AJ, Pendarvis K, Cooksey AM, Burgess SC, Rhoads DD. A proteome-based model for sperm mobility phenotype. Journal of Animal Science 2011;89(5) 1330-7.

[10] Bakst MR. Physiology and Endocrinology Symposium: Role of the oviduct in maintaining sustained fertility in hens. Journal of Animal Science 2011;89(5)1323-9.

[11] Perry MM, Waddington D, Gilbert AB, Hardie MA. Growth rates of the small yolky follicles in the ovary of the domestic fowl. IRCS Medical Science: Experimental Animals 1983;11(11/12) 979-80.

[12] Saito N, Sato K, Shimada K. Prostaglandin levels in peripheral and follicular plasma, the isolated theca and granulosa layers of pre- and postovulatory follicles, and the myometrium and mucosa of the shell gland (uterus) during a midsequence-oviposition of the hen (Gallus domesticus). Biology of Reproduction 1987;36(1) 89-96.

[13] Dick HR, Culbert J, Wells JW, Gilbert AB, Davidson MF. Steroid hormones in the postovulatory follicle of the domestic fowl (*Gallus domesticus*). Journal of Reproduction and Fertility 1978;53(1) 103-8.

[14] Hammond RW, Olson DM, Frenkel RB, Biellier HV, Hertenlendy F. Prostaglandins and steroid hormones in plasma and ovarian follicles during the ovulation cycle of

the domestic hen (*Gallus domesticus*). General and Comparative Endocrinology 1980;42(2) 195-202.

[15] Hertenlendy F, Biellier HV, Todd H. Effects of the egg cycle and the route of administration on prostaglandin-induced oviposition of hens and Japanese quail. Journal of Reproduction and Fertility 1975;44(3) 579-82.

[16] Johnson AL, Woods DC. Ovarian dynamics and follicle development. In: Jamieson BGM, editor. Reproductive Biology and Phylogeny of Birds.Enfield, New Hampshire: Science Publishers; 2007. p. 243-77.

[17] Wyburn GM, Johnston HS, Draper MH, Davidson MF. The fine structure of the infundibulum and magnum of the oviduct of *Gallus domesticus*. Quarterly Journal of Experimental Physiology 1970;55(3):213-32.

[18] Perry MM. Nuclear events from fertilisation to the early cleavage stages in the domestic fowl (*Gallus domesticus*). Journal of Anatomy 1987;150(1) 99-109.

[19] Birkhead TR, Sheldon BC, Fletcher F. A comparative study of sperm–egg interactions in birds. Journal of Reproduction and Fertility 1994;101(2) 353-61.

[20] Bakst MR, Howarth B, Jr. Hydrolysis of the hen's perivitelline layer by cock sperm in vitro. Biology of Reproduction 1977;17(3) 370-9.

[21] Okamura F, Nishiyama H. The passage of spermatozoa through the vitelline membrane in the domestic fowl, Gallus gallus. Cell and Tissue Research 1978;188(3) 497-508.

[22] Bakst MR, Wishart G, Brillard JP. Oviductal sperm selection, transport, and storage in poultry. Poultry Science Reviews 1994;5 117-43.

[23] Froman DP, Feltmann AJ, McLean DJ. Increased fecundity resulting from semen donor selection based upon in vitro sperm motility. Poultry Science 1997;77(1) 73-7.

[24] Bakst MR. Observations on the turkey oviductal sperm-storage tubule using differential interference contrast microscopy. Journal of Reproduction and Fertility 1992;95(3) 877-83.

[25] Schuppin GT, Van Krey HP, Denbow DM, Bakst MR, Meyer GB. Ultrastructural analyses of uterovaginal sperm storage glands in fertile and infertile turkey breeder hens. Poultry Science 1984;63(9) 1872-82.

[26] Bakst MR, Akuffo V. Alkaline phosphatase reactivity in the vagina and uterovaginal junction sperm-storage tubules of turkeys in egg production: Implication for sperm storage. British Poultry Science 2007;48(4) 515-8.

[27] Brillard JP. Sperm storage and transport following natural mating and artificial insemination. Poultry Science 1993;72(5) 923-8.

[28] Christensen VL, Bagley LG. Efficacy of fertilization in artificially inseminated turkey hens. Poultry Science 1989;68(5) 724-9.

[29] Bakst MR, Donoghue AM, Yoho DE, Moyle JR, Whipple SM, Camp MJ, et al. Comparisons of sperm storage tubule distribution and number in 4 strains of mature broiler breeders and in turkey hens before and after the onset of photostimulation. Poultry Science 2010;89(5) 986-92.

[30] Birkhead TR, Moller AP. Numbers and size of sperm storage tubules and the duration of sperm storage in birds: A comparative study. Biological Journal of the Linnean Society 1992;45(4):363-72.

[31] Brillard JP, Beaumont C, Scheller MF. Physiological responses of hens divergently selected on the number of chicks obtained from a single insemination. Journal of Reproduction and Fertility 1998;114(1) 111-7.

[32] Bakst MR. Oviducal sperm selection, transport, and storage in poultry: A review. Reproduction Fertility and Development 1993;5(6) 595-9.

[33] Blesbois E, Brillard JP. Specific features of *in vivo* and *in vitro* sperm storage in birds. Animal 2007;1(10):1472-81.

[34] Van Krey HP, Ogasawara FX, Pangborn J. Light and electron microscopic studies of possible sperm gland emptying mechanisms. Poultry Science 1967;46(1) 69-78.

[35] Fujii S. Histological and histochemical studies on the oviduct of the domestic fowl with special reference to the region of utero-vaginal junction. Archives of Histology and Cytology 1963;23(5) 447-9.

[36] Renden JA, May EB, Benoff FH. Histochemistry of uterovaginal sperm-host glands in Japanese quail (*Coturnix coturnix japonica*) with reference to the period of oviposition. Poultry Sci 1981;60(11) 2529-35.

[37] Blesbois E, Lessire M, Grasseau J, Hallouis JM, Hermier D. Effect of dietary fat on the fatty acid composition and fertilizing ability of fowl semen. Biology of Reproduction 1997;56(5) 1216-20.

[38] Surai PF. Natural Antioxidants in Avian Nutrition and Reproduction. Nottingham, UK: Nottingham University Press; 2002.

[39] Williams K, Frayne J, Hall L. Expression of extracellular glutathione peroxidase type 5 (GPX5) in the rat male reproductive tract. Molecular Human Reproduction 1998;4(9) 841-8.

[40] Catalá A. Lipid peroxidation modifies the picture of membranes from the "Fluid Mosaic Model" to the "lipid whisker model". Biochimie 2012;94(1) 101-9.

[41] Breque C, Surai P, Brillard JP. Roles of antioxidants on prolonged storage of avian spermatoza *in vivo* and *in vitro*. Molecular Reproduction and Development 2003;66(3) 314-23.

[42] Long C, Sonstegard TS, Long JA, van Tassell CP, Zuelke KA. Serial analysis of gene expression in turkey sperm storage tubules in the presence and absence of resident sperm. Biology of Reproduction 2003;69(2) 469-74.

[43] Foye-Jackson OT, Long JA, Bakst MR, Blomberg LA, Akuffo V, Silva VB, et al. Oviductal expression of avidin, avidin-related protein-2, and progesterone receptor in turkey hens in relation to sperm storage: Effects of oviduct tissue type, sperm presence, and turkey line. Poultry Science 2011;90(7) 1539-47.

[44] O'Malley BW, McGuire WL. Studies on the mechanism of action of progesterone in regulation of the synthesis of specific protein. Journal of Clinical Investigation 1968;47(3) 654-64.

[45] Korpela JK, Elo HA, Tuohimaa PJ. Aviadin induction by estrogen and progesterone in te immature oviduct of chicken, Japanese quail, duck, and gull. General and Comparative Endocrinology 1981;44(2) 230-2.

[46] Burke WH, Ogasawara FX. Presence of spermatozoa in uterovaginal fluids of the hen at various stages of the ovulatory cycle. Poultry Science 1969;48(2) 408-13.

[47] Compton MM, Van Krey HP, Siegel PB. The filling and emptying of the uterovaginal sperm-host glands in the domestic hen. Poultry Science 1978;57(6) 1696-700.

[48] Bushman AF, Van Krey HP, Denbow DM, Siegel PB. Effect of the ovulatory cycle on oviductal sperm storage in the domestic fowl. Theirogenology 1985;23(3) 473-9.

[49] Bakst MR. Duration of fertility of turkeys inseminated at different times after the onset of photostimulation. Journal of Reproduction and Fertility 1988;84(2) 531-7.

[50] Das SC, Nagasaka N, Yoshimura Y. Changes in the expression of estrogen receptor mRNA in the utero-vaginal junction containing sperm storage tubules in laying hens after repeated artifical insemination. Theriogenology 2006;64(4) 893-900.

[51] Yoshimura Y, Koike K, Okamoto T Immunolocalization of progesterone and estrogen receptors in the sperm storage tubules of laying and diethylstilbestrol-injected immature hens. Poultry Science 2000;79(1) 94-8.

[52] Ito T, Yoshizaki N, Tokumoto T, Ono H, Yoshimura Y, Tsukada A, et al. Progesterone is a sperm-releasing factor from the sperm-storage tubules in birds. Endocrinology 2011;152(10) 3952-62.

[53] Agre P, Sasaki S, Chrispeels MJ. Aquaporins: A family of water channel proteins. American Journal of Physiology Renal Physiology 1993;265(3) F461.

[54] Zaniboni L, Bakst MR. Localization of aquaporins in the sperm storage tubules in the turkey oviduct. Poultry Science 2004;83(7) 1209-12.

[55] Froman DP, Bowling ER, Wilson JL. Sperm mobility phenotype not determined by sperm quality index. Poultry Science 2003;82(3) 496-502.

[56] Froman DP. Effect of sperm mobility phenotype on fertility, sperm competition, and in vivo sperm storage in the domestic fowl. Journal of Dairy Science 93[Suppl. 1], 504. 2010.

[57] Brillard JP, Galut O, Nys Y. Possible causes of subfertility in hens following insemination near the time of oviposition. British Poultry Science 1987;28(2) 307-18.

[58] Stephens RE, Prior G. Dynein from serotonin-activated cilla and flagella: Extraction characteristics and distinct sites for cAMP-dependent protein phosphorylation. Journal of Cell Science 1992;103(4):999-1012.

[59] Holm L, Ridderstrale Y, Knutsson PG. Localisation of carbonic anhydrase in the sperm storing regions of the domestic hen. Cell Tissues Organs 1996;156(4):253-60.

[60] Holm L, Wishart GJ. The effect of pH on the motility of spermatoza from chicken, turkey and quail. Animal Reproduction Science 1998;54(1):45-54.

[61] Freedman SL, Akuffo VG, Bakst MR. Evidence for the innervations of sperm storage tubules in the oviduct of the turkey (*Meleagris gallopavo*). Reproduction 2001;121(5): 809-14.

[62] Bakst MR, Akuffo V. Serotonin localization in the turkey vaginal but not sperm storage tubule epithelia. Journal of Avian Biology 2008;39(3):348-54.

[63] Froman DP, Bowling ER, Wilson JL. Sperm mobility phenotype not determined by sperm quality index. Poultry Science 2003;82(3):496-502.

[64] Froman DP, Engel HN. Alteration of the spermatozoal glycocalyx and its effect on duration of fertility in the fowl (*Gallus domesticus*). Biology of Reproduction 1989;40(3):615-22.

[65] Froman DP, Thursam KA. Desialylation of the rooster sperm's glycocalyx decreases sperm sequestration following intravaginal insemination of the hen. Biology of Reproduction 1994;50(5):1094-9.

[66] Steele MG, Wishart GJ. Demonstration that the removal of sialic acid from the surface of chicken spermatozoa impedes their transvaginal migration. Theriogenology 1996;46(6):1037-44.

[67] Pelaez J, Long JA. Characterizing the glycocalyx of poultry spermatozoa: I. Identification and distribution of carbohydrate residues using flow cytometry and epifluorescence microscopy. Journal of Andrology 2007;28(2):342-52.

[68] Robertson L, Wishart GJ, Horrocks AJ. Identification of perivitelline N-linked glycans as mediators of sperm-egg interaction in chickens. Journal of Reproduction and Fertility 2000;120(2):397-403.

[69] Birkhead TR, Brillard JP. Reproductive isolation in birds: postcopulatory prezygotic barriers. Trends in Ecology & Evolution 2007;22(5):266-72.

[70] Steele MG, Meldrum W, Brillard JP, Wishart GJ. The interaction of avian spermatozoa with the perivitelline layer in vitro and in vivo. Journal of Reproduction and Fertility 1994;101(3):599-603.

[71] Howarth B. Carbohydrate involvement in sperm-egg interaction in the chicken. Journal of Receptor Research 1992;12(2):255-65.

[72] Horrocks AJ, Stewart JM, Jackson L, Wishart GJ. Induction of acrosomal exocytosis in chicken spermatozoa by inner perivitelline-derived N-linked glycans. Biochemical and Biophysical Research Communications 2000;278(1):84-9.

[73] Koyanagi F, Masuda S, Nishiyama H. Acrosome reaction to cock spermatoza incubated with the perivitelline layer of the hen's ovum. Poultry Science 1988;67(12): 1770-4.

[74] Bakst MR, Howarth B, Jr. The fine structure of the hen's ovum at ovulation. Biology of Reproduction 1977;17(3):361-9.

[75] Wasserman PM, Jovine L, Litscher ES. A profile of fertilization in mammals. Nature Cell Biology 2001;3(2):E59-64.

[76] Stepinska U, Olszanska B. DNase I and II present in avian oocytes: A possible involvement in sperm degradation at polyspermic fertilisation. Zygote 2003;11(1): 35-42.

[77] Stepinska U, Bakst MR. Fertilization. In: Jamieson BGM, editor. Reproductive Biology and Phylogeny of Birds. Enfield, New Hampshire: Science Publishers; 2007. p. 553-87.

[78] Wishart GJ. Quantitative aspects of sperm:egg interaction in chickens and turkeys. Animal Reproduction Science 1997;48(1):81-92.

[79] Bellaris R, Harkness M, Harkness RD. The vitelline membrane of the hen's egg: A chemical and electron microscopal study. Journal of Ultrastructure Research 1963;8(3):339-59.

[80] Bramwell RK, Howarth B, Jr. Preferential attachment of cock spermatozoa to the perivitelline layer directly over the germinal disc of the hen's ovum. Biology of Reproduction 1992;47(5):1113-7.

[81] Wishart GJ. Regulation of the length of the fertile period in the domestic fowl by numbers of oviducal spermatozoa, as reflected by those trapped in laid eggs. Journal of Reproduction and Fertility 1987;81(2):495-9.

[82] Brillard JP, Antoine H. Storage of sperm in the uterovaginal junction and its incidence on the numbers of spermatoza present in the perivitelline layer of hen's eggs. British Poultry Science 1990;31(3):635-44.

[83] Wishart GJ. Quantitative aspects of sperm:egg interaction in chickens and turkeys. Animal Reproduction Science 1997;48(1):81-92.

[84] Malecki IA, Rybnik PK, Martin GB, Malecki I, Glatz P. Artificial insemination technology for ratites: A review. Australian Journal of Experimental Biology 2008;48(10): 1284-92.

[85] Bakst MR, Cecil HC. Gross appearance of turkey cloacae before and after single or multiple manual semen collections. Poultry Science 1983;62(4):683-9.

[86] Haugland RP. Handbook of Fluorescent Probes and Research Products. 9th ed. Eugene, Oregon: Molecular Probes, Inc.; 2002.

[87] Froman DP, McLean DJ. Objective measurement of sperm motility based upon sperm penetration of Accudenz®. Poultry Science 1996;75(6):776-84.

[88] Froman DP. Application of the sperm mobility assay to primary broiler breeder stock. Journal of Applied Poultry Research 2006;15(2):280-6.

[89] Bakst MR, McGary S, Estevez I, Knapp T. Use of nonsettable eggs to evaluate turkey hen fertility. Journal of Applied Poultry Research 2002;11(4):402-5.

[90] Brillard JP, Bakst MR. Quantification of spermatozoa in the sperm-storage tubules of turkey hens and the relation to sperm numbers in the perivitelline layer of eggs. Biology of Reproduction 1990;43(2):271-5.

[91] Bramwell RK, Marks HL, Howarth B. Quantitative determination of spermatozoa penetration of the perivitelline layer of the hen's ovum as assessed on oviposited eggs. Poultry Science 1995;74(11):1875-83.

[92] Donoghue AM. The effect of twenty-four hour *in vitro* storage on sperm hydrolysis through the perivitelline layer of ovipositioned turkey eggs. Poultry Science 1996;75(8):1035-8.

[93] Lake, PE. Historical perspective of artificial insemination technology. In: Bakst MR and Wishart GJ, editors. Proceedings - First International Symposium on the Artifical Insemination of Poultry. Savoy, Illinois: Poultry Science Association; 1995. p. 1-20